Anti-Inflammatory Cookbook

Detox and Rejuvenate Your Body by Strengthening Your Immune System

Laura Ruiz

Disclaimer Notice:

Please note the information contained within this document is for educational and entertainment purposes only. All effort has been executed to present accurate, up-to-date, and reliable, complete information. No warranties of any kind are declared or implied. Readers acknowledge that the author is not engaging in the rendering of legal, financial, medical, or professional advice. The content within this book has been derived from various sources. Please consult a licensed professional before attempting any techniques outlined in this book.

By reading this document, the reader agrees that under no circumstances is the author responsible for any losses, direct or indirect, which are incurred as a result of the use of the information contained within this document, including, but not limited to, — errors, omissions, or inaccuracies.

Table of Contents

Anti-Inflammatory Cookbook

BREAKFAST

Chive Smoked Salmon Toast

Prep time: 5 minutes

Cooking time: 0 minutes

Servings: 1

Ingredients:
- ½ tsp dried chives
- ¼ tsp garlic-infused oil
- 2 tbsp lactose-free cream cheese
- 1 slice gluten-free bread, toasted
- ¾ oz. plain smoked salmon
- Kosher salt & ground black pepper to taste

Instructions:
1. In a small bowl, combine the cream cheese, garlic-infused oil, and dried chives.
2. Top the bread with the cream cheese mixture and sprinkle some salt and pepper on top of the salmon before serving.

Nutritional Information: Calories: 307; Carbs: 29g; Fat: 15g; Protein: 14g

Basmati Rice Gruel

Prep time: 5 minutes
Cooking time: 20 minutes
Servings: 1
Ingredients:
- 2 cups warm water
- 1 tsp salt
- 1 cup basmati rice
- 2 tsp ground cinnamon
- 1/3 tsp ground nutmeg
- 2 tbsp pure maple syrup
- 1 can of unsweetened coconut milk

Instructions:
1. Rice and water should be brought to a boil in a medium saucepan. Give it a minute to simmer. 2.Add the unsweetened coconut milk, unsweetened maple syrup, cinnamon, and nutmeg. With the lid on, cook the rice for 20 minutes while stirring occasionally. Serve!

Nutritional Information: Calories: 130; Carbs: 12g; Fat: 5g; Protein: 8g

Crustless Bacon Zucchini Quiche

Prep time: 10 minutes
Cooking time: 30 minutes
Servings: 8

Ingredients:

- 2 large zucchinis, grated
- 1/2 cups (6 oz) grated cheddar
- 2 tbsp canola oil
- 6 large eggs, lightly beaten
- Salt & freshly ground black pepper to taste

Instructions:

1   Grease a 9-inch quiche dish, line it with parchment paper, and preheat the oven to 350°F.

2   Use paper towels to cover a platter.

3   Add the bacon to a pan that has not yet been heated, and cook for 10 minutes over medium heat, turning often, until crispy. Transfer to a plate lined with paper towels to drain any extra oil.

4   After the bacon has cooled enough to handle, cut it into little pieces.

5   In a big bowl, combine the bacon, zucchini, cheese, oil, and eggs. Add salt and pepper to taste.

6   Put the mixture in a baking dish and bake for 20 to 25 minutes, or until it is firm and browned.

7   Let it cool before serving.

Nutritional Information: Calories: 258; Carbs 25g; Fat 5.6g; Protein 4g

Eggs in a Basket

Prep time: 10 minutes

Cooking time: 3 minutes

Servings: 4

Ingredients:

- 2 eggs
- 2 slices of sourdough bread, toasted if desired
- 2 tsp butter or ghee
- Water, as needed
- Dash of paprika (optional)

Instructions:

1. Fill a deep pan with three to four inches of water and bring it to a boil over high heat. Separately breaking each egg (into two little cups)s, gently placing them in the boiling water, and covering them right away.
2. Cook the eggs for 3 minutes after turning off the heat, or until they are just barely runny.
3. After each bread slice has been spread with butter or ghee, pierce it in the middle.
4. Using a slotted spoon, put each fried egg into the hole of one slice of bread. Serve with a sprinkle of paprika on top.
   Nutritional Information: Calories: 311; Carbs: 16g; Fat: 7.1g; Protein: 44 g

Cucumber Avocado Toast

Prep time: 5 minutes

Cooking time: 0 minutes

Servings: 1

Ingredients:

- 1 English cucumber, thinly sliced
- Kosher salt & black pepper to taste
- ¼ tsp paprika
- ¼ tsp Halaby pepper
- ¼ small avocado pitted
- ½ tsp lime juice
- 1 Gluten-free bread slice, toasted

Instructions:

1.   Combine the cucumber slices with a sprinkle of salt, pepper, paprika, and Halaby pepper in a medium bowl.

2.   In another dish, mash the quartered avocado with a fork and add salt and pepper to taste before incorporating the lime juice.

3.   Evenly distribute the mashed avocado over the bread. Serve the avocado with the spicy cucumber slices on top.

Nutritional Information: Calories: 130; Carbs: 24g; Fat: 3g; Protein: 2g

Strawberries and Cream Oatmeal

Prep time: 5 minutes
Cooking time: 5 minutes
Servings: 1
Ingredients:

- 1 cup quick cooking rolled oats
- 2 cups water
- 1 banana, peeled & sliced
- 5 strawberries, sliced
- 2 oz coconut milk

Instructions:

1. In a skillet, mix the water and rolled oats. After letting it come to a boil, reduce the heat to low and simmer for another five minutes.

2.The strawberries and bananas should be combined in a bowl. Stir thoroughly after adding the cooked oats and coconut milk before serving.

Nutritional Information: Calories: 195; Carbs 21g; Fat 3.2g; Protein 6.2g

Banana with Chia Seeds Pancakes

Prep time: 10 minutes
Cooking time: 4 minutes
Servings: 2

Ingredients:

- 2 eggs
- 1 banana, mashed
- 1 tbsp chia seeds
- 1 tbsp brown rice flour
- 1 tsp vanilla extract
- 1 tsp cinnamon
- Nonstick cooking spray

Instructions:

1.The eggs are beaten in a medium bowl. Banana, chia seeds, brown rice flour, vanilla, and cinnamon should all be added to the bowl and mixed well.

2. Spray the bottom of a large pan with cooking spray and preheat it over medium-high heat.

3. Spoon each pancake with two heaping tablespoons of batter, and cook for one to two minutes, or until bubbles start to appear on the top. 4. Once the bottoms are golden brown, flip the

pancakes over and cook for an additional 1 to 2 minutes. Serve

Nutritional Information: Calories: 168; Carbs: 9g; Fat: 8g; Protein: 9g

Parsley Egg Scramble

Prep time: 10 minutes
Cooking time: 4 minutes
Servings: 4
Ingredients:

- 1 bunch parsley, finely chopped
- 8 eggs
- 1/4 tsp salt
- 1/4 tsp freshly ground black pepper
- 1 tbsp extra-virgin olive oil
- Water, as needed

Instructions:

1. Bring to a boil over high heat in a medium saucepan with enough water. Cook the parsley for one minute after adding it. Rinse with cold water after a thorough draining.
2. In a medium bowl, combine the eggs, cooked parsley, salt, and pepper.
3. Heat the oil in a large nonstick pan over medium heat. The eggs should be cooked to your preference after 2 to 3 minutes of gentle whisking after adding the eggs. Serve immediately.
   Nutritional Information: Calories: 186; Carbs 18.7g; Fat 9g; Protein 7.2g

Breakfast Chickpea Flour Flatbread

Prep time: 10 minutes
Cooking time: 5 minutes
Servings: 4
Ingredients:

- 1½ cups chickpea flour
- ½ tsp ground turmeric
- ½ tsp sea salt
- ½ tsp ground black pepper
- 2 tbsp + 2 tsp extra-virgin olive oil
- 1½ cups water

Instructions:

1.   In a bowl, stir together the chickpea flour, turmeric, salt, and black pepper. Stir well before adding water and 2 tablespoons of olive oil. until smooth, combine, and stir.

2.   In an 8-inch nonstick pan, heat 2 tablespoons of olive oil over medium-high heat until it shimmers.

3.   Pour half a cup of the mixture into the skillet and swirl it around to coat the bottom with the mixture.

4.   Cook for 5 minutes, or until crispy and gently browned. About halfway through the cooking process, flip the flatbread. The leftover mixture should be used again. Slice and warmly serve.

Nutritional Information: Calories: 207; Carbs: 20.7g; Fat: 10.2g; Protein: 7.9g

Oat Cereal and Spiced Pumpkin Quinoa

Prep time: 10 minutes
Cooking time: 20 minutes
Servings: 4

Ingredients:

- 1 cup unsweetened pumpkin puree
- 4 cups water
- Pinch of salt
- ¾ tsp ground cinnamon
- 1 cup quick oats
- 1 cup quinoa, rinsed
- ½ cup walnut pieces

Instructions:

1.In a large saucepan over medium-high heat, bring the pumpkin, water, salt, and cinnamon to a boil, stirring regularly. Add the quinoa and oats.

2.The oats and quinoa should be cooked after around 15 minutes of cooking at medium heat with regular stirring.

3.Add the walnuts after turning the heat off. Serve right away.

Nutritional Information: Calories: 120; Carbs: 19g; Fat: 4g; Protein: 4g

Chicken and Spinach Omelet

Prep time: 10 minutes
Cooking time: 25 minutes
Servings: 2

Ingredients:

- 4 large eggs
- ¼ cup roughly chopped basil
- ¼ cup roughly chopped flat-leaf parsley
- Salt & freshly ground black pepper to taste
- 1 tbsp canola oil
- ½ cup shredded cooked chicken
- A small handful of baby spinach leaves, rinsed, dried, & chopped
- ½ red bell pepper, diced
- ¼ cup (1 oz) grated cheddar

Instructions:

1. In a medium bowl, combine the eggs, basil, and parsley, season with salt and pepper.
2. In a medium frying pan over medium heat, heat the oil. Add the egg mixture, tilting the pan topcoat the bottom.
3. Cook until the top is nearly set. Lift the edges of the omelet gently with a spatula or pancake turner, then shake it free.
4. Cover one-half of the omelet with the chicken, spinach, bell pepper, and cheese. To enclose the filling, fold the other half over the top.
5. Heat the filling and cheese just enough to begin melting. Before serving, remove the omelet from the pan and split it in half.

Nutritional Information: Calories: 343; Carbs: 4g; Fat: 23g; Protein: 29g

Sweet Potato Spinach Frittata

Prep time: 10 minutes
Cooking time: 30 minutes
Servings: 4
Ingredients:
- 1/2 tbsp butter
- 2 small, sweet potatoes, cut into 1/2-inch cubes
- 2 cups baby spinach leaves
- 1 cup crumbled strong blue cheese
- 8 eggs, lightly beaten
- Salt & freshly ground black pepper to taste

Instructions:
1. Set the oven's temperature to 350°F.
2. Over medium heat, melt the butter in a 7-inch skillet, ideally one with an ovenproof handle.
3. Include the cubes of sweet potato and simmer for 10 minutes, or until they are soft and golden-brown.
4. In a bowl, gently mix the eggs, spinach, and blue cheese. Pour over the sweet potatoes and bake for 20 to 25 minutes, or until the sweet potatoes are crisp.
5. Take it out of the oven and let it cool before slicing. Serve.
   Nutritional Information: Calories: 317; Carbs: 16g; Fat: 8.6g; Protein: 25g

Mini Banana Pancakes

Prep time: 10 minutes

Cooking time: 6 minutes

Servings: 4

Ingredients:

- 2 small bananas, peeled
- 2 large eggs
- 2 tbsp gluten-free all-purpose flour
- ½ tsp ground cinnamon
- ¼ tbsp ground nutmeg
- 1 tbsp brown sugar
- ¼ tsp baking powder
- 1/8 tsp salt

Instructions:

1. Peel the bananas and mash them till smooth in a big dish. Prior to adding the flour, cinnamon, and nutmeg, thoroughly mix the eggs.
2. Include salt, baking soda, and brown sugar.
3. Scoop a batter onto a nonstick frying pan that has been heated over medium heat. Cook the batter until it begins to bubble slightly on top.
4. Turn the pancake over and continue cooking it until the second side is golden brown. Serve!
   Nutritional Information: Calories 96; Carbs 17.3g; Fat 2.5g; Protein 2.3g

PB Banana Overnight Oats

Prep time: 10 minutes + chilling time
Cooking time: 5 minutes
Servings: 4

Ingredients:

- 2 cups gluten-free rolled oats
- 4 tsp chia seeds
- 2 medium bananas, mashed
- 4 tbsp natural and no sugar added peanut butter
- 2 cups unsweetened almond milk
- 1 tsp ground cinnamon

Instructions:

1. Combine the cinnamon, almond milk, peanut butter, bananas, chia seeds, and oats in a glass dish. Combine well by tossing, then wrap in plastic.
2. Place in the fridge and serve right away the next morning.
   Nutritional Information: Calories: 359; Protein: 19g; Carbs: 60g; Fat: 14g

Olive Frittata and Mozzarella Tomato

Prep time: 10 minutes
Cooking time: 20 minutes
Servings: 4
Ingredients:

- 6 eggs
- 1 medium tomato, diced
- ½ cup black olives
- ¼ cup chopped scallions
- ½ cup shredded Mozzarella cheese
- Pinch of sea salt
- Freshly ground black pepper, to taste

Instructions:

1   Set the oven to 400 degrees.
2   In a large bowl, whisk the eggs with a little water. Place aside.
3   Arrange the cheese, tomato, olives, scallions, and olives in a cast-iron pan or 9-by-9-inchbaking dish. Add salt and pepper to the dish after adding the eggs.
4   Bake the eggs until they are set, about 20 to 25 minutes. Before cutting the frittata, let it cool for five minutes.

Nutritional Information: Calories: 144; Carbs: 4g; Fat: 10g; Protein: 11g

Breakfast Muesli

Prep time: 10 minutes

Cooking time: 15 minutes

Servings: 6

Ingredients:

- 5 cups gluten-free cornflakes
- 1 ½ cups quinoa puffs
- 7 tbsp dried shredded coconut
- 4 tbsp pumpkin seeds
- 15 banana chips, crushed
- 6 tbsp olive oil
- 1/3 cup brown sugar

Instructions:

1   Set the oven to 300 Fahrenheit.

2   Put the cornflakes in a plastic bag and use a rolling pin to smash them.

3   Combine the banana chips, coconut, pumpkin seeds, coconut puffs, cornflakes, and quinoa puffs in a bowl. Brown sugar and olive oil are combined. combine well after mixing.

4   Distribute the mixture on a baking sheet that has been covered with parchment paper. To ensure consistent cooking, bake for 15 minutes in the oven while tossing every 10 minutes.

5   Allow the muesli to cool after cooking it before storing it in an airtight container.

Nutritional Information: Calories 464; Carbs 56.3g; Fat 19.5g; Protein 11.2g

Quinoa Porridge with Berries

Prep time: 10 minutes

Cooking time: 20 minutes

Servings: 2

Ingredients:

- ½ cup quinoa
- ¾ cup coconut milk
- ¼ tsp ground cinnamon
- 4 tsp pure maple syrup
- 1 cup fresh berries of your choice
- 1 tsp oil
- 1 cup water

Instructions:

1. Put the quinoa in a strainer and give it a minimum of two minutes' worth of rinsing under running water.
2. Add oil to the location in the pan. Toast the quinoa over medium heat or until it becomes brown.
3. Pour a cup of water on top and heat until boiling. 15 minutes of simmering should make it frothy. Reintroduce the quinoa to the pan after draining any extra water.
4. Add the maple syrup, cinnamon, and coconut milk. Give the porridge five minutes to cook.

   Just before serving, pour the berries in.

   Nutritional Information: Calories 441; Carbs 46.8g; Fat 26.5g; Protein 8.6g

Cinnamon Banana Crepes

Prep time: 10 minutes
Cooking time: 1-2 minutes
Servings: 4
Ingredients:

- ½ cup gluten-free flour
- 2 medium bananas
- ¼ tsp sugar-free pure vanilla extract
- 1 cup almond milk, separated
- ¼ tsp ground cinnamon
- 4 tsp extra virgin olive oil, separated

Instructions:

1. In a pan over medium heat, warm 2 tablespoons of olive oil.
2. In the meantime, use an electric mixer to thoroughly combine the almond milk, bananas, cinnamon, vanilla, and flour in a glass dish for 45 seconds.
3. Swirl a batter into the pan to ensure a uniform distribution. Turn to the other side after heating for 30 seconds or until the edges start to darken.
4. After 30 seconds of cooking, move the dish to a serving tray. Use tin foil to enclose it. Repeat with the remaining batter after heating 2 teaspoons in the skillet. Serve.
   Nutritional Information: Calories: 165; Carbs: 17g; Fat: 11g; Protein: 3g

LUNCH

Bok Choy Tuna Salad

Prep time: 10 minutes

Cooking time: 0 minutes Servings: 2-4

Ingredients:

- 5 oz canned tuna, strained
- ½ tsp crushed tarragon
- 1 ½ tsp fresh lemon juice
- 2/3 cup low fodmap mayonnaise
- 1 tsp Dijon mustard
- ¾ cup bok choy stems, chopped
- Flaky sea salt & ground black pepper to taste

Instructions:

1.Scrape the tuna that has been drained into a big basin. Mix in the bok choy stems, mayonnaise, lemon juice, crushed tarragon, and mustard.

2. Add black pepper and flaky sea salt to taste. Serve!

Nutritional Information: Calories: 71; Carbs: 5g; Fat: 5g; Protein: 3g

Brown Rice & Vegetable Bowl

Prep time: 10 minutes

Cooking time: 0 minutes

Servings: 4

Ingredients:

- 3 cups low-FODMAP vegetables, roasted
- ½ cup spring onions, green parts only, chopped
- 3 tbsp parsley, finely chopped
- 2 cups arugula, chopped
- 2 cups cooked brown rice
- 3 tbsp roasted pumpkin seeds
- 3 tbsp feta, crumbled
- Kosher salt & ground black pepper to taste
- ½ tsp brown sugar
- 3 tbsp olive oil
- 1½ tbsp lemon juice
- 1½ tbsp balsamic vinegar

Instructions:

1. Combine the cooked rice, pumpkin seeds, feta, spring onions, parsley, and arugula in a large bowl.
2. Add salt and pepper as desired. Place aside.
3. In a small bowl, combine the sugar, balsamic vinegar, lemon juice, and olive oil. Serve the salad after drizzling the dressing over it.

   Nutritional Information: Calories: 260; Carbs: 36g; Fat: 9g; Protein: 9g

Pineapple Shrimp Fajitas

Prep time: 10 minutes
Cooking time: 15 minutes
Servings: 4

Ingredients:

- 1 pound shrimp, cleaned & deveined
- 2 tbsp olive oil
- 2 tbsp lime juice
- 1 tbsp fresh chives
- 2 tbsp fresh cilantro
- 1 cup pineapple chunks
- 2 cups red bell peppers, sliced
- 2 cups cooked brown rice
- 8-10 corn tortillas

Instructions:

1. In a bowl, combine the olive oil, lime juice, cilantro, and chives. After adding, coating, and setting aside for 5 minutes, add the shrimp.
2. Set a grill, either inside or outside, to medium heat. Place pineapple chunks in between rows of shrimp on the skewers.
3. Thread the shrimp onto the skewers and grill for 3 to 4 minutes on each side, or until the shrimp is cooked through.
4. In the meantime, coat your pan with cooking spray and sauté the peppers for 3–4 minutes over medium heat, or until firm and tender.
5. Take the shrimp off the grill and serve it with the brown rice that has been cooked and the sautéed peppers. Serve!

   Nutritional Information: Calories: 219; Carbs: 28.5g; Fat: 1.5g; Protein: 22g

Orange Chicken

Prep time: 10 minutes
Cooking time: 27 minutes
Servings: 8

Ingredients:

- 1 ½ pounds chicken thighs, skinless & boneless
- 1 tsp olive oil
- ½ tsp pepper
- ½ tsp ground coriander
- 1 tsp ground ginger
- 1 tsp salt

For the sauce:

- 2 tbsp arrowroot powder
- 1 tbsp fish sauce
- 1 tbsp vinegar
- ¼ cup butter
- ¼ cup coconut amino
- 1 orange juice & zest

Instructions:

1. Oven temperature: 425 °F.
2. Combine the sauce's components in a small bowl and whisk to combine.
3. In a large bowl, combine the coriander, ginger, pepper, and salt. Add the chicken and generously sprinkle the spice mixture over it.
4. In a large pan, heat the oil to a medium-high temperature. Cook the chicken for 3–4 minutes after adding it. Cook the chicken for one minute after flipping it. The chicken should be moved to a baking dish.

5. Add the sauce mixture to the pan and heat for one to two minutes, or until it thickens.
6. Cover the chicken with the sauce and bake it for 15-20 minutes in a preheated oven. Enjoy after serving.
   Nutritional Information: Calories: 328; Carbs: 11.1g; Fat: 14.6g; Protein: 35.6g

Gingered Carrot Soup

Prep time: 15 minutes
Cooking time: 30 minutes Servings: 4-6
Ingredients:
- 2 tbsp butter
- 1 lb. carrots, peeled & diced
- 2 tbsp fresh grated ginger
- ½ tsp salt
- ½ tsp black pepper
- ½ tsp cinnamon
- ½ tsp nutmeg
- 4 cups onion-free chicken or vegetable broth
- 1 cup cooked pumpkin, mashed
- 1 cup almond milk
- ¼ cup walnuts, chopped
- ¼ cup fresh parsley, chopped

Instructions:
1. Pour butter into a big soup pot.
2. Add the carrots, salt, black pepper, cinnamon, and nutmeg to the heated butter and sauté for 5 to 7 minutes, turning periodically, until the carrots are soft.
3. Include the ginger and simmer for a further 1-2 minutes. After adding the broth, the heat should be set to medium-high.
4. Bring the broth to a boil, then reduce the heat and simmer it for 15 minutes.
5. Include the pumpkin in the soup and purée with an immersion blender until smooth. Add almond milk and stir until the desired consistency is achieved.
6. Cook for another five minutes on low heat. Serve with walnuts and fresh parsley as garnish.
Nutritional Information: Calories 253; Carbs 48g; Fat 10.2g; Protein 10.4g

Lemon-Butter Tilapia with Almonds

Prep time: 10 minutes

Cooking time: 5 minutes

Servings: 4

Ingredients:

- 4 oz tilapia fillets
- 1¼ cup butter, cubed
- ¼ cup white wine or onion-free chicken broth
- 2 tbsp lemon juice
- ¼ cup sliced almonds
- ½ tsp salt
- ¼ tsp pepper
- 1 tbsp olive oil

Instructions:

1. Sprinkle some salt and pepper on the fish.
2. Cook the fish for two to three minutes on each side in hot oil in a big skillet. Keep warm and set aside.
3. Combine the wine, lemon juice, and butter in the same pan. Until the butter has melted, cook and stir.
4. Before serving, spread the butter mixture over the fish and top with almonds.
   Nutritional Information: Calories 269; Carbs 1g; Fat 19g; Protein 22g

Quinoa & Rice Khichri

Prep time: 10 minutes
Cooking time: 28 minutes
Servings: 4

Ingredients:

- ½ red bell pepper, chopped
- 1 carrot, peeled & diced
- 2 cups vegetable broth
- 1 cup uncooked quinoa
- 1 tsp turmeric powder
- ½ tsp ground cumin
- 1 cup brown rice, cooked
- ¼ cup parsley, chopped
- 2 tbsp garlic-infused olive oil
- Himalayan salt & ground black pepper to taste

Instructions:

1. Combine the red pepper, carrot, vegetable broth, quinoa, turmeric, and cumin in a large saucepan over medium-high heat.
2. After the majority of the liquid has decreased, let the quinoa simmer for 25 minutes.
3. Include the parsley, garlic-infused oil, and cooked brown rice. To ensure that everything is well cooked and mixed, stir for 2 to 3 minutes. 4. Add salt and pepper as desired. Serve warm.
Nutritional Information: Calories: 96; Carbs: 12g; Fat: 5g; Protein: 2g

Italian Herb-Style Ribbon Pasta

Prep time: 10 minutes
Cooking time: 25-30 minutes
Servings: 4
Ingredients:

- 12 oz. gluten-free ribbon pasta
- ¼ cup garlic-infused olive oil
- 1 cup fresh parsley, chopped
- 8 oz. canned fire-roasted red peppers, seeded & chopped
- Sea salt & ground black pepper to taste

Instructions:

1. Place a big saucepan on the stovetop and add salted water. Bring to a boil. Pasta should be added and cooked until al dente while stirring often to avoid sticking.
2. Place a colander over a sink and pour the cooked pasta through it to drain.
3. Add the oil, parsley, and red peppers to the drained pasta in a large serving dish. Before serving, season with salt and pepper to taste.
Nutritional Information: Calories: 210; Carbs: 43g; Fat: 1g; Protein: 7g

Rustic Potato Soup

Prep time: 15 minutes
Cooking time: 45 minutes
Servings: 6

Ingredients:

- ¼ pound bacon, diced
- 6 medium potatoes, cut into cubes
- 2 cups carrots, diced
- 3 cups Swiss chard, chopped
- ½ tsp salt
- ½ tsp black pepper
- 1 tsp dried thyme
- ¼ cup fresh parsley
- 2 tbsp fresh chives
- 5 cups low-fodmap chicken or vegetable broth
- ½ cup fresh grated parmesan cheese
- ½ cup almond milk

Instructions:

1. Place the bacon in a large stockpot or soup pot and cook it over medium-high heat, turning often, until it is crisp and browned.
2. Add the carrots and simmer for a further 4–5 minutes while stirring. Add the potatoes, salt, black pepper, thyme, and Swiss chard.
3. After one or two minutes, add the broth and bring it to a boil. The potatoes and carrots should be soft after 20 minutes of simmering at low heat.
4. Transfer half of the soup to a blender, if required, working in batches. Transfer the mixture back into the soup pot with the remaining liquid after blending until smooth.

5.Combine the almond milk, parmesan cheese, chives, and parsley. Before serving, simmer for another 5–10 minutes over low heat.

Nutritional Information: Calories 167; Carbs 48g; Fat 10.2g; Protein 14g

Herbed Tilapia with Lime

Prep time: 10 minutes
Cooking time: 14 minutes
Servings: 2
Ingredients:

- 1 tbsp olive oil
- 1/8 tsp each thyme & dried basil
- 1/4 tsp salt
- 2 (6-oz) tilapia fillets
- Juice of 1/2 a lime

Instructions:

1. Heat the olive oil in a pan over medium heat.
2. Evenly season both sides of the fillets with salt, thyme, and basil. They should be placed in the pan and cooked for 5 to 7 minutes on each side, or until done.
3. Before serving, arrange the fillets on plates and top with lime juice.
   Nutritional Information: Calories: 342; Carbs: 22g; Fat: 12g; Protein: 23g

Asian Chicken and Rice Bowl

Prep time: 15 minutes

Cooking time: 10 minutes

Servings: 4

Ingredients:

- 1-pound boneless skinless chicken breast
- 1 ½ cup red bell pepper, sliced
- 6 cups fresh spinach, chopped
- ½ cup water chestnuts
- 1 tbsp sesame oil
- ¼ cup soy sauce
- 1 tbsp fresh grated ginger
- ½ tsp black pepper
- ½ cup peanuts, chopped
- 1 tbsp sesame seeds
- 3 cups hot cooked basmati rice

Instructions:

1. Heat the sesame oil in a pan over medium-high heat. Black pepper is then added, and the chicken is cooked for 2 minutes.
2. Include the red bell pepper and simmer for an additional two to three minutes. Water chestnuts, spinach, and freshly grated ginger should all be added.
3. Stir in the soy sauce, then cook the chicken and spinach together until the spinach wilts.4. Spoon the hot, cooked basmati rice over the chicken and vegetable combination. Before serving, garnish with chopped peanuts and sesame seeds.
   Nutritional Information: Calories: 534; Carbs: 10.8g; Fat: 18.5g; Protein: 5.8g

Coconut Zucchini Soup

Prep time: 10 minutes
Cooking time: 28 minutes
Servings: 4

Ingredients:

- 1 zucchini, chopped
- 1 bell pepper, chopped
- 2 carrots, chopped
- 1 cup of coconut milk
- 1 cup of water
- 1 tbsp olive oil

Direction:

1. In a pan over medium heat, warm the olive oil. When the veggies are ready, add them to the pan and simmer for a further 7–8 minutes.
2. Include the coconut milk, mix well, and simmer for 5 minutes at medium heat. Cook for 15 minutes on low heat after adding the water.
3. Season the soup with salt and pepper and use an immersion blender to puree the soup until it is smooth. Enjoy after serving.
   Nutritional Information: Calories: 202; Carbs: 10.8g; Fat: 18g; Protein: 2.8g

Spiced Quinoa with Almonds & Feta

Prep time: 15 minutes

Cooking time: 17 minutes

Servings: 4

Ingredients:

- 1 ½ cups quinoa, rinsed
- 1/2 tsp turmeric
- 1 tbsp olive oil
- 1 tsp ground coriander
- 1/2 cup almonds, toasted & flaked
- 1 cup feta cheese, crumbled
- 1/2 lemon juice
- Handful parsley, chopped

Instructions:

1. Add the spices to a skillet with hot oil and cook for one minute.
2. After the second minute, stir in the quinoa. Cook for 15 minutes after adding 2 1/2 cups of boiling water.
3. After letting it cool, mix in the other ingredients. Stir thoroughly, then plate.

   Nutritional Information: Calories: 321; Carbs: 5g; Fat: 15g; Protein: 3g

Beef & Zucchini Stir-Fry

Prep time: 10 minutes
Cooking time: 15 minutes
Servings: 4

Ingredients:

- 1 tsp toasted sesame oil
- 1 tsp fresh ginger, grated
- 1 tbsp dark brown sugar
- 1 tbsp oyster sauce
- 3 tbsp soy sauce
- 8 oz cooked Asian rice noodles
- 2 tbsp garlic-infused olive oil
- 1 lb. beef sirloin fillets, sliced across the grain
- 2 medium carrots, peeled & diced
- 1 cup zucchini, chopped

Instructions:

1. In a small bowl, combine the ginger, dark brown sugar, oyster sauce, and soy sauce with the toasted sesame oil. While assembling the remainder of the meal, cover the sauce.
2. Place the cooked noodles in a large bowl, add 1 tablespoon of garlic-infused oil, and toss to combine.
3. Add the beef strips to the remaining olive oil that has been heated in a large pan over medium high heat.
4. Stir until the strips are well cooked, about 4–5 minutes. Put the scraped meat in a basin and keep it heated.
5. Put the pan back on the heat and cook the carrots and zucchini for 3 to 4 minutes, or until they are soft to the fork.
6. Add the steak and cooked noodles, then toss for a couple of minutes in the sauce to cover everything. Serve right away.

Nutritional Information: Calories: 190; Carbs: 9g; Fat: 4g; Protein: 20g

Cheesy Swiss Chard Wraps

Prep time: 10 minutes
Cooking time: 15 minutes
Servings: 8

Ingredients:

- 1 tbsp. garlic-infused olive oil
- 8 oz. Swiss chard, rinsed & chopped
- 8 large soft corn wraps
- 2 cups baby tomatoes, halved
- 2 cups mozzarella cheese, shredded

Instructions:

1. In a large pan, heat the oil over medium-high heat. Add the Swiss chard, tossing for 5 minutes, or until it has shrunk in size by half. Place aside.
2. Add one corn wrap and put the heat back on the pan. Add 1/4 of the tomato halves, enough cooked chard, and cheese to the wrap's top, then top with another wrap.
3. Firmly press it into the pan. The wraps should be cooked for 6 minutes with a cover on, turning once. With the remaining wraps and ingredients, repeat the procedure.
4. Arrange the cooked wraps on a serving tray, then cut them into pieces to serve.
   Nutritional Information: Calories: 65; Carbs: 13g; Fat: 1g; Protein: 6g

Deep Fried Eggplant Rolls

Prep time: 15 minutes

Cooking time: 6 minutes Servings: 4-6

Ingredients:

- 2 large eggplants, trimmed & cut lengthwise into ¼-inch-thick slices
- 1 tsp salt
- 1 cup ricotta cheese
- 4 oz goat cheese, shredded
- ¼ cup finely chopped fresh basil
- ½ tsp freshly ground black pepper
- Olive oil spray

Instructions:

1. Place the salt-seasoned eggplant slices in a colander. Set aside for 15 to 20 minutes.
2. In a large bowl, mix the ricotta, goat cheese, basil, and black pepper. Place aside.
3. After using paper towels to dry the eggplant slices, gently spray them with olive oil.
4. Lightly spritz a sizable pan with olive oil and heat it over medium heat.
5. Place the sliced eggplant in the pan and cook for 3 minutes on each side, or until golden-brown.
6. Transfer the food off the stove and let it cool for five minutes on a platter lined with paper towels.
7. Arrange the eggplant slices on a level surface and sprinkle a spoonful of the prepared cheese mixture on top of each piece. Serve them right after rolling them.
   Nutritional Information: Calories: 254; Carbs: 18.6g; Fat: 14.9g; Protein: 15.3g

Maple -Bourbon Baked Salmon

Prep time: 10 minutes + marinating time
Cooking time: 15 minutes
Servings: 6
Ingredients:

- 1½ pounds salmon fillet
- 2 tbsp 100% pure maple syrup
- 1 tbsp olive oil
- 1 tbsp olive oil
- ¼ tsp sweet smoked paprika
- ½ tsp salt
- 2 tbsp bourbon

Instructions:

1. In a bowl, mix the bourbon, salt, paprika, oil, and maple syrup. Turn the salmon skin-side down after placing it skin-side up in the marinade. Well-covered, marinate for 8 to 10 hours.
2. Set the oven to 400 degrees. A baking dish big enough to hold the fish should have its bottom and half of its sides covered with foil.
3. Arrange the salmon in the pan, skin-side down. After 10 minutes, baste the fish with the hot pan juices and bake for another 15 minutes, or until the salmon flakes opaquely with a fork.
   Nutritional Information: Calories: 407; Carbs: 6g; Fat: 35g; Protein: 7g

Roasted Vegetables with Feta

Prep time: 10 minutes
Cooking time: 30 minutes
Servings: 4

Ingredients:

- 1 zucchini, chopped
- 1 red bell pepper, seeded & chopped
- 1 yellow bell pepper, seeded & chopped
- 2 carrots, peeled & chopped
- 2 tbsp olive oil
- 1 tbsp dried rosemary
- ½ cup feta cheese
- Salt & pepper to taste

Instructions:

1. Line a baking sheet with parchment paper and preheat the oven to 350 degrees Fahrenheit.
2. Arrange all the veggies in a baking dish; sprinkle with olive oil; and season to taste with salt, pepper, and rosemary.
3. Bake for 30 minutes in the oven. For even cooking, be sure to jiggle the baking sheet every ten minutes.
4. After the veggies have finished cooking, arrange them on a serving platter and top with feta.
   Serve.

   Nutritional Information: Calories 135; Carbs 6.8g; Fat 11g; Protein 3.6g

Spinach Zucchini Soup

Prep time: 10 minutes
Cooking time: 25 minutes
Servings: 6

Ingredients:

- 6 medium zucchinis, chopped
- 1 cup coconut milk
- 1 cup baby spinach
- 4 cups water
- Salt & pepper to taste

Instructions:

1. In a large saucepan, combine water and zucchini, simmer over medium heat. Make it boil. Set the temperature to low and simmer for 25 minutes.
2. Remove and then include spinach and coconut milk. Season the soup with salt and pepper after using an immersion blender to puree it until smooth. Enjoy after serving.
   Nutritional Information: Calories: 129; Carbs: 10.1g; Fat: 9.9g; Protein: 3.6g

DINNER

Gourmet Zucchini Angel-Hair "Pasta"

Prep time: 10 minutes
Cooking time: 0 minutes
Servings: 4
Ingredients:

- 1 large or 2 medium green or yellow zucchinis
- 12 black olives, pitted
- 1 cup tiny broccoli florets
- 4 sun-dried tomatoes, sliced
- 1 to 2 fresh tomatoes, finely diced
- 1 tbsp balsamic vinegar
- 1 clove of garlic, minced
- 3 oyster mushrooms, sliced
- 1 /4 tsp each sea salt & cracked pepper, or to taste
- 1 /8 tsp oregano, or to taste

Instructions:

1. Slice, grate, or spiralize the zucchini into thin strips before placing it on a large serving platter. 2. Combine the olives, broccoli, and both kinds of tomatoes with the vinegar and garlic in a mixing bowl. Add the salt, pepper, and oregano to the mushrooms along with the oil mixture.

3. Place the zucchini "pasta" on a plate and top it with the olive-mushroom mixture.

Nutritional Information: Calories: 215; Carbs: 26g; Fat: 21g; Protein: 15g

Roasted Pepper Pasta

Prep time: 10 minutes
Cooking time: 10 minutes
Servings: 4
Ingredients:

- 4 cups gluten-free pasta, cooked
- 3 tbsp parmesan cheese, grated
- 3 tbsp fresh basil leaves, chopped
- 1 tbsp tapioca starch
- 1 cup unsweetened almond milk
- 2 tbsp olive oil
- ¼ cup pumpkin puree
- 2 cups red bell peppers, roasted
- Salt to taste

Instructions:

1. In a blender, combine the roasted bell peppers, parmesan cheese, basil leaves, tapioca starch, almond milk, and olive oil. Process until smooth.
2. Transfer the sauce to a large pan and warm over medium-high heat.
3. Give the sauce a good stir and heat it until it slightly thickens. Toss the cooked spaghetti with the sauce. Serve after adding salt.

   Nutritional Information: Calories: 308; Carbs: 47.5g; Fat: 10g, Protein: 7g

Lemon Butter Shrimp Over Vegetable Noodles

Prep time: 10 minutes

Cooking time: 12 minutes

Servings: 4

Ingredients:

- 1 lb. shrimp, cleaned & deveined
- ¼ cup butter
- 1 tbsp lemon juice
- 1 tbsp capers
- ½ tsp salt
- ½ tsp black pepper
- 4 cups zucchini, spiral sliced into noodles

Instructions:

1. Bring to a boil some water that has been mildly salted. Cook the spiralized zucchini in the water for two to three minutes.
2. To stop the cooking of the zucchini, carefully remove it from the cooking water and place it in a dish of cold water. Before draining, let it settle for a few seconds.
3. In a pan over medium heat, melt the butter. Add salt and black pepper to the shrimp and drizzle with lemon juice.
4. Add the capers and shrimp to the skillet with the butter. Cook for two to three minutes on each side, or until fully done.
5. Transfer the cooked zucchini noodles to serving dishes after tossing them in the heated butter in the pan.
   Nutritional Information: Calories: 431; Carbs: 7.1g; Fat: 20.4g; Protein: 53.4g

Pasta With Salmon and Dill

Prep time: 10 minutes
Cooking time: 15 minutes
Servings: 3

Ingredients:

- 1 packet of gluten-free pasta
- 1 tbsp olive oil
- 1/3 oyster mushrooms, sliced
- zest of 1 lime
- ½ smoked salmon
- 3 cups baby spinach
- 1 cup low fodmap chicken stock
- 1 tbsp corn flour
- 1 cup almond milk
- 1 bunch of dill

Instructions:

1. Add the mushrooms to a skillet with the oil already heated over medium heat and cook for 2 to 3 minutes.
2. Include the fish, chicken stock, lime juice, lime zest, and baby spinach leaves.
3. Stir the milk and corn flour together in a bowl until combined. Add the cooked spaghetti and dill to the pan after pouring in this mixture.
4. Stir to evenly coat the pasta. Add grated cheese to the serving dish.
   Nutritional Information: Calories: 162; Carbs: 18g; Fat: 3.1g; Protein: 9.3g

Stuffed Chicken Breasts

Prep time: 10 minutes
Cooking time: 16 minutes
Servings: 2

Ingredients:

- ¼ cup Greek yogurt
- ¼ cup spinach, thawed & drained
- ½ cup artichoke hearts, thinly sliced
- ½ cup mozzarella cheese, shredded
- 1½ lb. chicken breasts
- 2 tbsp olive oil
- 4 oz cream cheese
- Sea salt & pepper, to taste

Instructions:

1. Thickness the chicken breasts to approximately an inch. Make a "pocket" into each side with the use of a sharp knife. Salt and pepper the breasts, then put them aside.
2. Combine the spinach, artichokes, cream cheese, yogurt, mozzarella, salt, and pepper in a medium bowl.
3. Insert the mixture into each breast's compartment and set aside.
4. In a big skillet over medium heat, warm the oil. Turn off the heat after cooking each breast for8 minutes on each side. Serve.

Nutritional Information: Calories: 885, Carbs: 10g, Fat: 64.48g, Fiber: 2.6g, Protein: 65.28g

Spicy Fried Shrimp & Broccoli

Prep time: 10 minutes
Cooking time: 5-10 minutes
Servings: 6
Ingredients:

- 1 tsp brown sugar
- 1 tsp cayenne pepper
- 1 tsp corn flour
- 2 tbsp low-sodium, low-fodmap soy sauce
- ½ cup chicken broth
- 2 tbsp garlic-infused olive oil
- 2 tbsp fresh ginger, peeled & finely chopped
- 2 cups small broccoli florets
- 1 lb. large shrimp, peeled & deveined
- 2 tsp toasted sesame oil
- ¼ cup spring onions, chopped (green parts only)

Instructions:

1. In a medium bowl, combine the sugar, cayenne pepper, corn flour, soy sauce, and chicken broth. Place aside.
2. Fry the ginger for one minute in the oil in a big pan over medium heat.
3. Increase the heat to medium-high and stir-fry the broccoli for 2 minutes, or until it is well browned. When the shrimp start to turn pink, add them and toss for approximately 30 seconds. 4. Add the stock and mix while cooking the sauce for approximately a minute. Before serving, take off the skillet and toss in the sesame oil and spring onions.
Nutritional Information: Calories: 259; Carbs: 6g; Fat: 9g; Protein: 30g

Pecan Salmon Fillets

Prep time: 10 minutes
Cooking time: 15 minutes
Servings: 6

Ingredients:

- 3 tbsp olive oil
- 3 tbsp mustard
- 5 tsp maple syrup
- 1 cup pecans, chopped
- 6 salmon fillets, boneless
- 1 tbsp lemon juice
- 3 tsp parsley, chopped
- Salt & pepper to the taste

Instructions:

1. In a bowl, mix together the oil, mustard, and honey.
2. Add the parsley and pecans to another bowl.
3. After seasoning the salmon with salt and pepper, place the fillets on a baking sheet covered with parchment paper, brush the fillets with the honey-mustard mixture, and then sprinkle the pecan mixture on top.
4. Bake for 15 minutes in a 400°F oven. Serve the mixture between plates with a sprinkle of lemon juice.
   Calories: 282; Carbs: 20.9g; Fat: 15.5g; Protein: 16.8g

Ratatouille Casserole

Prep time: 10 minutes
Cooking time: 25 minutes
Servings: 8
Ingredients:

- 5 tbsp olive oil
- 1 eggplant, sliced
- 1 zucchini, sliced
- 1 red bell pepper, seeded & sliced
- 1 can of diced tomatoes
- 2 tbsp chopped thyme
- 2 tbsp chopped oregano
- 2 tbsp chopped rosemary
- ½ cup white wine
- 3 basil leaves, torn
- 4 parsley leaves, torn
- 1 cup grated Parmigiano cheese
- 2 cups Gruyere cheese
- Salt & pepper to taste

Instructions:

1. Oil a casserole dish and preheat the oven to 375°F.
2. In a pan over medium-high heat, add the oil and wilt the eggplant, zucchini, and red bell pepper. Add salt and pepper to taste. The vegetables should be put in a casserole dish.
3. Combine the tomatoes, white wine, thyme, oregano, and rosemary in a bowl.
4. Pour it on top of the veggies and garnish with parsley and basil. Add Gruyere and Parmigiano cheeses on top.
5. After 20 minutes of baking, serve.
   Nutritional Information: Calories 298; Carbs 6.1g; Fat 24.6g; Protein 15g

Chicken Curry

Prep time: 10 minutes
Cooking time: 12 minutes
Servings: 2
Ingredients:

- 1 tbsp coconut oil
- 1 red bell pepper, diced
- 1 spring onion, green parts only, chopped
- 3 large skinless chicken breasts, sliced into small cubes
- 2 tbsp turmeric powder
- 1 tbsp curry powder
- 2 tins of unsweetened coconut milk
- Himalayan salt & ground black pepper to taste
- 2 cups basmati rice, cooked for serving

Instructions:

1. In a large pan over medium-high heat, melt the coconut oil. Add the bell pepper and spring onion. The vegetables should be fork-tender after frying for 3 to 5 minutes.
2. Add the chicken cubes and stir. Fry for 7 minutes, or until the chicken is fully cooked.
3. Combine turmeric, curry powder, and unsweetened coconut milk; add salt and pepper to taste.
4. Place the cooked basmati rice on a plate and top with the hot curry.

Nutritional Information: Calories: 160; Carbs: 18g; Fat: 2g; Protein: 26g

Worcestershire Pork Chops

Prep time: 10 minutes

Cooking time: 13 minutes

Servings: 3

Ingredients:

- 2 tbsp Worcestershire sauce
- 8 oz pork loin chops
- 1 tbsp lemon juice
- 1 tsp olive oil

Instructions:

1. In a bowl, combine the Worcestershire sauce, lemon juice, and olive oil. Brush the sauce mixture on both sides of the pork loin chops.
2. Set the grill's temperature to 395 °F. The pork chops should be cooked for 5 minutes on the grill.
3. After turning the pork chops over, brush the opposite side with the leftover sauce mixture. Serve the meat after another 7–8 minutes of grilling.
   Nutritional Information: a3aCalories: 267; Carbs: 2.1g; Fat: 20.4g; Protein: 17g

Spinach and Pancetta Pasta

Prep time: 10 minutes

Cooking time: 30 minutes

Servings: 6

Ingredients:

- 1-pound gluten-free pasta
- 2 tbsp garlic-infused olive oil, + additional for serving (optional)
- 8 oz thinly sliced lean pancetta
- 5 cups of baby spinach leaves
- 1/4 cup pine nuts
- 1/2 cup grated Parmesan
- Salt & freshly ground black pepper

Instructions:

1. In a big pot of boiling water, cook the pasta until just al dente, as directed on the box. Drain and then add back to the saucepan. cover to stay warm.
2. Heat the last tablespoon of oil in a large pan. Add the pancetta, spinach, and pine nuts after cooking until the pine nuts are browned and the spinach is wilted.
3. Over medium heat, toss the pasta with the Parmesan until the cheese has melted.
4. Add salt and pepper to taste and, if you'd like, a little extra oil. Serve.

   Nutritional Information: Calories:367; Carbs:25g; Fat: 29g; Protein:24g

Coconut Chicken Rice Noodle

Prep time: 10 minutes
Cooking time: 10 minutes
Servings: 4
Ingredients:

- 1 package rice noodle
- 2 tbsp coconut oil
- 1 lb. chicken breasts
- 1 zucchini, sliced
- 1 bell pepper, seeded & sliced
- 2 carrots, peeled & sliced
- 1 can of coconut milk
- Salt & pepper to taste

Instructions:

1. Prepare the rice noodles as directed on the packet. drain, then set apart.
2. In a large pan over medium heat, heat the coconut oil. Fry the chicken breasts for 3 minutes on each side, or until golden brown.
3. Add the carrots, zucchini, and bell pepper, season with salt and pepper, to taste. For one minute, stir.
4. Pour the coconut milk in. Simmer for 6 minutes with the cover on the pan. After thoroughly tossing in the cooked noodles, serve.
   Nutritional Information: Calories 415; Carbs 22.5g; Fat 13.9g; Protein 19.6g

Shrimp with Beans

Prep time: 10 minutes
Cooking time: 10 minutes
Servings: 4
Ingredients:

- 1 lb. shrimp, peeled and deveined
- 2 tbsp soy sauce
- 2 tbsp olive oil
- salt to taste
- ½ lb. green beans, washed & trimmed

Instructions:

1. In a pan, heat the oil to a medium-high temperature. Sauté the beans for 5–6 minutes, or until they are soft. Turn off the heat and put the pan aside.
2. Include the shrimp and cook it for two to three minutes on each side in the same pan. Soy sauce and the beans should be added back to the pan.
3. Continue to boil the shrimp while stirring often. Serve after adding salt.
   Nutritional Information: Calories: 217; Carbs: 6.4g; Fat: 9g; Protein: 27.4 g

Potato Curry in Coconut Milk

Prep time: 10 minutes
Cooking time: 14 minutes
Servings: 7

Ingredients:

- 2 tbsp garlic-infused olive oil
- 1 tbsp fresh ginger, peeled & crushed
- 1 cup carrots, peeled & chopped
- 1 tsp ground cumin
- 2 tsp turmeric powder
- 28 oz canned tomatoes
- 1 cup raw quinoa
- 3 cups vegetable broth
- ½ cup unsweetened coconut milk
- 1½ cups waxy potatoes, boiled & cubed
- Kosher salt & ground black pepper to taste

Instructions:

1. Place a large cast-iron saucepan over medium heat, then add the oil, ginger, and carrots that have been diced. Carrots should be cooked through after 5 to 10 minutes of frying.
2. Include the turmeric and cumin powders. Stir for one to two minutes to let the flavors mingle.
3. Add the quinoa, tomatoes, and vegetable broth. The quinoa should soften after 5 minutes of simmering.
4. Include the potato cubes and coconut milk. To fully reheat the potatoes, stir for 1-2 minutes.

Before serving, season with a little salt and pepper to taste.

Nutritional Information: Calories: 79; Carbs: 18g; Fat: 0g; Protein: 3g

FISH & SEAFOODS

Seafood in Coconut Sauce

Prep time: 10 minutes
Cooking time: 6 minutes
Servings: 4
Ingredients:

- 1 tbsp coconut oil
- 1 tsp minced ginger
- 1 cup mussel meat
- ½ cup crab meat, shredded
- ½ cup prawns, peeled & deveined
- 1 cup coconut cream
- 1 lemongrass stalk
- Salt & paper to taste

Instructions:

1. Heat the oil and sauté the ginger in a large skillet for a minute. Stir in the mussels, crab meat, and prawns.
2. Add in the coconut cream and lemongrass. Allow to cook for 6 minutes or until the prawns are done.
   Nutritional Information: Calories 341; Carbs 18.7g; Fat 25.3g; Protein 15.7g

England Shrimp Boil

Prep time: 10 minutes

Cooking time: 8 minutes

Servings: 8

Ingredients:
- 2 tbsp olive oil
- 1 tbsp fennel seed
- 1 tbsp mustard seed
- ½ tsp red pepper flakes
- 3 (12-oz) bottles of beer
- 1 lemon, quartered
- 3 lb. fresh shrimps head off, and shells on
- ½ cup unsalted butter salt & pepper to taste

Instructions:
1. Heat the oil in a large saucepan before adding the fennel and mustard seeds and toasting them. Salt and pepper to taste, then incorporate the red pepper flakes.
2. After adding the beer, add the lemon wedges to the saucepan. Add the shrimp, then cook for four minutes.
3. Empty the liquid from the shrimp and drain them. Before serving, arrange the shrimp on a dish and dot them with butter.
   Nutritional Information: Calories 186; Carbs 0.9g; Fat 9.2g; Protein 23.7g

Shrimp Cakes with Tangy Paprika Aioli

Prep time: 10 minutes

Cooking time: 8 minutes

Servings: 4

Ingredients:

- 1-pound large raw shrimp, peeled, deveined, & rinsed
- 1 large egg, beaten
- 2 scallions (green part only), diced
- 2 tbsp freshly squeezed lemon juice
- 1 tbsp Dijon mustard
- ¾ tsp cayenne pepper
- 2 cups gluten-free bread crumbs
- 1/8 tsp sea salt
- 1 cup mayonnaise
- Juice & grated zest of 1 lime
- ½ tsp paprika
- 2 tbsp olive oil

Instructions:

1. Pulse the shrimp in a food processor's bowl until it is finely chopped.
2. Include the egg, the scallion greens, the lemon juice, the Dijon mustard, and the 1/4 teaspoon cayenne. Shortly pulse to mix. To blend, add 1 cup of the bread crumbs and pulse just once.
3. Create 8 cakes out of the mixture. Incorporate the cakes with the last cup of bread crumbs. Place on a baking sheet covered with paper, then chill for ten minutes.
4. While the shrimp cakes are cooling, combine the remaining 1/2 teaspoon cayenne, mayonnaise, lime juice, lime zest, paprika, and sea salt in a small dish. Place aside.
5. Heat the oil to shimmering in a large nonstick pan over medium-high heat.

6. Fry the cakes in batches until they are evenly golden brown, approximately 4 minutes on each side. Serve the cakes with the aioli on top.

Nutritional Information: Calories: 660; Carbs: 24g; Fat: 32g; Protein: 35g

Shrimp with Lime and Cheddar Tacos

Prep time: 10 minutes

Cooking time: 22 minutes

Servings: 4

Ingredients:

- 2 tbsp garlic oil
- Juice of 1 lime
- ¼ tsp cayenne pepper
- 1-pound large raw shrimp, peeled, deveined, & rinsed
- 8 scallions
- 8 (6-inch) corn tortillas
- 4 oz Cheddar cheese, shredded
- ¼ cup chopped fresh cilantro

Instructions:

1. In a medium bowl, combine the cayenne, lime juice, and garlic oil. Stir in the shrimp, then set it aside for ten minutes.
2. Lightly oil the grill and preheat it to medium heat. The shrimp are skewered and then placed on the grill. The shrimp should be cooked for approximately 5 minutes on each side until pink.
3. Place the scallions on the grill and cook them for approximately 3 minutes each side, flipping them regularly, until they are just beginning to burn.

4. Trim the white portion of the scallions and throw it away. Scallion greens should be cut in half lengthwise. The tortillas should be grilled on the grill for approximately 3 minutes each side, flipping them periodically.
5. To assemble, wrap the heated corn tortillas in the shrimp, scallion greens, Cheddar cheese, and cilantro. Serve.

Nutritional Information: Calories: 424; Carbs: 29g; Fat: 20g; Protein: 36g

Snapper with Tropical Salsa

Prep time: 15 minutes
Cooking time: 8 minutes
Servings: 4

Ingredients:

- 2 tbsp extra-virgin olive oil
- 1 pound snapper, quartered
- 1 tsp sea salt, divided
- 1/8 tsp freshly ground black pepper
- 1 papaya, chopped
- 1 cup chopped pineapple
- 1 jalapeño pepper, seeded & minced
- 1 tbsp chopped fresh cilantro leaves
- Juice of 1 lime

Instructions:

1. In a large nonstick pan, heat the olive oil over medium-high heat until it shimmers.
2. Sprinkle 12 teaspoons each of salt and pepper on the snapper. When the fish is opaque, add it to the pan and cook for approximately 4 minutes on each side.
3. Gently combine the papaya, pineapple, cilantro, jalapeno, lime juice, and remaining 1/2 teaspoon salt in a medium bowl. Serve the snapper with the salsa on top.
Nutritional Information: Calories: 236; Carbs: 14g; Fat: 8g; Protein: 27g

Cacciuto

Prep time: 10 minutes
Cooking time: 8 minutes
Servings: 4

Ingredients:

- 1 tbsp olive oil
- 1 small fennel bulb, peeled & sliced thinly
- 2 medium carrots, peeled & chopped
- 1 cup white wine
- 4 small filleted white fish
- 1 cup prawn meat
- Lemon cut into wedges
- Salt & pepper to taste

Instructions:

1.In a saucepan with a medium burner, heat the oil, then sauté the carrots and fennel bulb for 5 minutes, or until they are soft.

2. Include the white wine and simmer for three minutes. Add the fish fillet and prawn flesh, and season to taste with salt and pepper. Lemon wedges should be served.

Nutritional Information: Calories 282; Carbs 17.1g; Fat 7.9g; Protein 36.3g

Creamy Smoked Salmon Pasta

Prep time: 10 minutes

Cooking time: 7 minutes

Servings: 4

Ingredients:

- 2 tbsp garlic oil
- 6 scallions, green parts only, chopped
- 2 tbsp capers, drained
- 12 oz smoked salmon, flaked
- ¾ cup unsweetened almond milk
- 2 tbsp chopped fresh dill
- 1/8 tsp freshly ground black pepper
- 8 oz gluten-free pasta, cooked according to the package directions and drained

Instructions:

1. In a large nonstick pan, heat the garlic oil over medium-high heat until it shimmers. Add the capers and scallions. While stirring, cook for 2 minutes.
2. Include the fish and cook for another two minutes. Add the pepper, dill, and almond milk by stirring. 3 minutes of simmering Serve after tossing the heated pasta.
   Nutritional Information: Calories: 287; Fat: 6g; Carbs: 35g; Protein: 23g

Salmon Fillet with Carrot Ribbon

Prep time: 10 minutes
Cooking time: 25 minutes
Servings: 2

Ingredients:

- 2 (6-oz) salmon fillets
- Sea salt, to taste
- Freshly ground black pepper, to taste
- 1-pound whole carrots, skin peeled
- Nonstick cooking spray
- 1 tsp extra-virgin olive oil, + extra for the grill
- 1 tbsp fresh parsley, loosely chopped

Instructions:

1. For 10 to 15 minutes, heat up an outside grill on medium-high. Salt and pepper the fillets after patting them dry with paper towels.
2. Cover the grill with cooking spray. Each slice of salmon should be placed skin-side up, fillet side down. Cook the first side for 4 more minutes after flipping after 6 minutes of cooking.
3. While the salmon is cooking, peel the carrots into ribbons using a vegetable peeler.
4. Toss the carrots with the olive oil, salt, and parsley in a small bowl. Over the carrot ribbons, place the cooked salmon.
   Nutritional Information: Calories: 477; Carbs: 23g; Fat: 22g; Protein: 38g

Steamed Mussels with Saffron-infused Cream

Prep time: 10 minutes
Cooking time: 11 minutes
Servings: 4

Ingredients:

- 2 tbsp olive oil
- 1 tbsp Garlic Oil (here)
- 1 large bulb fennel, thinly sliced
- 1 cup dry white wine
- Large pinch saffron threads
- ¾ tsp salt
- ¾ cup heavy cream
- ¼ tsp freshly ground pepper
- 4 pounds cultivated mussels, rinsed well
- 2 tbsp chopped fresh flat-leaf parsley

Instructions:

1. In a stockpot, warm the olive oil and garlic oil over medium heat.
2. Add the fennel and simmer, stirring regularly, for approximately 5 minutes, or until tender. Bring to a boil after adding the salt, wine, and saffron. Add the mussels, pepper, and cream by stirring.
3. Cook the mussels under cover for approximately 6 minutes, or until they all open. Provide the mussels and broth in dishes with the parsley on top.
   Nutritional Information: Calories: 599; Carbs: 24g; Fat: 26g; Protein: 55g

Breaded Fish Fillets with Spicy Pepper Relish

Prep time: 10 minutes
Cooking time: 15 minutes
Servings: 4

Ingredients:

- 2 cups gluten-free bread crumbs
- 1¼ tsp sea salt, divided
- 1 tsp dried thyme
- 1/8 tsp freshly ground black pepper
- 2 eggs, beaten
- 1 tbsp Dijon mustard
- 1 pound cod, cut into 8 pieces
- 1 red bell pepper, chopped
- 2 tbsp capers, drained & rinsed
- 1 jalapeño pepper, minced
- Juice of 1 lime
- ¼ tsp red pepper flakes

Instructions:

1. Turn on the oven at 425 F.
2. Combine the bread crumbs, 1 teaspoon salt, pepper, and thyme in a small bowl.
3. Stir together the eggs and mustard in a separate small dish.
4. To coat the fish, dip it into the egg mixture and the breading mixture. On a baking sheet with a nonstick rim, put the fish.
5. Bake the fish for approximately 15 minutes, or until the crust is brown.
6. Combine the bell pepper, capers, jalapenos, lime juice, red pepper flakes, and the last 1/4 teaspoon of salt in a small bowl. Serve the fish with the relish on top.

Nutritional Information: Calories:209; Carbs: 13g; Fat: 3g; Protein: 30g

Seafood Adobo

Prep time: 10 minutes

Cooking time: 6 minutes

Servings: 4

Ingredients:

- 1 tbsp olive oil
- 1 medium red pepper, diced
- 1 tbsp adobo seasoning
- 2 cups blend of calamari, scallops, and shrimps
- 1/3 cup green olives, chopped
- Juice from ½ lemon
- Salt & pepper to taste

Instructions:

1. In a pan, heat the oil over medium heat. For 30 seconds, sauté the red pepper with the adobo spice.
2. Add the fish and green olives and stir. Lemon juice should be added, and salt and pepper should be added to taste.
3. It takes 6 minutes to cook the seafood to perfection.
   Nutritional Information: Calories 122; Carbs 14.6g; Fat 5.9g; Protein 2.7g

Sherry and Butter Prawns

Prep time: 10 minutes

Cooking time: 5 minutes

Servings: 4

Ingredients:

- 1½ pounds king prawns, peeled & deveined
- 2 tbsp dry sherry
- 1 tsp dried basil
- 1/2 tsp mustard seeds
- 1 ½ tbsp fresh lemon juice
- 1 tsp cayenne pepper, crushed
- 1/2 stick butter at room temperature

Instructions:

1. Combine the cayenne, basil, mustard seeds, lemon juice, and prawns in a bowl with the dry sherry. In your refrigerator, let it marinade for a full hour.
2. In a frying pan, melt the butter over medium-high heat while basting the meat with the saved marinade. Add salt and pepper according to taste.
   Nutritional Information: Calories 294; Carbs 3.6g; Fat 14.3g; Protein 34.6g

Grilled Halibut

Prep time: 10 minutes
Cooking time: 8 minutes
Servings: 1
Ingredients:

- 1 (12-oz) halibut fillet
- 2 tbsp lemon juice
- A dash of red pepper flakes
- Chopped parsley for garnish
- Salt & pepper to taste

Instructions:

1. Combine the halibut with all the other ingredients in a dish, leaving out the parsley. Marinate in the refrigerator for approximately an hour.
2. The grill should be at medium-high heat. Halibut should be placed on a hot grill rack and cooked for 4 minutes on each side or until flaky.
3. Garnish with parsley prior to serving.

Nutritional Information: Calories 679; Carbs 10.2g; Fat 47.7g; Protein 51.6g

Campfire Salmon

Prep time: 10 minutes
Cooking time: 15 minutes
Servings: 2

Ingredients:

- 2 oz salmon fillets
- 1 tbsp butter, melted
- 2 tbsp lemon juice
- 2 lemon wedges
- 1 tbsp minced fresh basil
- 1/8 tsp salt
- 1/8 tsp pepper

Instructions:

1. Place each fillet, skin side down, on a 12-inch square piece of heavy-duty foil.
2. Mix the melted butter, basil, lemon juice, salt, and pepper in a bowl. Drizzle over the salmon and seal the foil packets tightly.
3. Fold the foil around the fish, sealing it tightly.
4. Cook on a grill for 10–15 minutes.
5. Serve the fish in foil packets on serving plates with lemon wedges.
   Nutritional Information: Calories 274; Carbs 1g; Fat 19g; Protein 24g

Thai Coconut with Spinach Cod

Prep time: 10 minutes
Cooking time: 10 minutes
Servings: 2

Ingredients:

- 1 pound cod fillets
- Pinch of sea salt
- Freshly ground black pepper, to taste
- 1½ tsp coconut oil
- ⅓ cup canned coconut milk
- 1 tsp curry powder
- ½ tsp ground turmeric
- 1 cup fresh spinach
- Freshly squeezed lime juice (optional)

Instructions:

1. Add salt and pepper to both sides of the fish.
2. In a big skillet over medium heat, warm the oil. Cook the fish for one minute after adding it to the pan.
3. In a small bowl, combine the curry powder, turmeric, and coconut milk. The mixture should be added to the fish-filled skillet, covered, and cooked for 5 minutes.
4. After flipping the fish, add the spinach to the pan. The fish should be done after 4 minutes of cooking under cover.
5. Turn off the heat and add a squeeze of lime juice to the skillet (if using).
   Nutritional Information: Calories: 310; Carbs: 4g; Fat: 12g; Protein: 41g

Crusted Potato Flakes Cod Fillet

Prep time: 10 minutes
Cooking time: 8 minutes
Servings: 2
Ingredients:
- 1 cup rice flour
- 1 egg, lightly beaten
- 1 cup mashed potato flakes
- 1 pound cod fillets
- ½ tsp sea salt
- ½ tsp freshly ground black pepper
- 2 tbsp extra-virgin olive oil

Instructions:
1. Place the mashed potato flakes in one medium bowl, the beaten egg in another, and the rice flour in a third medium bowl.
2. Dip each cod fillet in the rice flour, then the egg, and then the mashed potato flakes, one at a time. The fillets should be salted and peppered.
3. In a large pan over medium-high heat, warm the olive oil. The fillets should be pan-fried for 4 minutes on each side, or until browned.
   Nutritional Information: Calories: 493; Carbs: 36g; Fat: 19g; Protein: 46g

Poached Red Snapper with Tomato Sauce

Prep time: 10 minutes
Cooking time: 8 minutes
Servings: 2

Ingredients:

- 1 can of diced tomatoes
- ¼ cup white wine
- ½ cup water
- 12 oz red snapper fillets
- 1 tsp salt
- Freshly ground black pepper, to taste
- ½ cup fresh basil leaves

Instructions:

1. In a medium pan over high heat, bring the water, wine, and tomatoes (with their juices) to aboil.
2. In the meantime, salt and pepper the fish on both sides.
3. Lower the heat to medium and add the fish to the pan, being sure to completely cover it with liquid.
4. Poach the fish for 8 to 10 minutes, or until it is well cooked, while covering the pan. At the very end of poaching the fish, stir in the basil.
   Nutritional Information: Calories: 276; Carbs: 8g; Fat: 3g; Protein: 45g

SOUPS, STEWS & SALADS

Italian Wedding Soup

Prep time: 15 minutes
Cooking time: 50 minutes
Servings: 2
Ingredients:

- 12 oz lean ground turkey or beef
- 1 large egg
- 2 tbsp quick-cooking oats
- 1 tbsp grated Parmesan cheese, + additional for garnish if desired
- ½ tsp dried basil
- 2 tsp garlic-infused olive oil
- 1½ quarts low-fodmap chicken or beef stock
- 2 medium carrots, diced
- ½ cup uncooked brown rice
- 4 cups tightly packed chopped kale
- ½ tsp salt, or more if needed
- ¼ tsp freshly ground black pepper

Instructions:

1. In a medium mixing bowl, combine the turkey, egg, oats, Parmesan, and basil. Make 1-inchballs using your hands or a little scoop.
2. In a large pan over medium heat, warm the oil until aromatic. The meatballs should be browned on all sides for 10 to 12 minutes, or until the middle is no longer pink. If necessary, drain any excess grease.
3. In a 4-quart pot, bring the stock to a boil. In a mixing dish, combine rice and carrots.

4. Cook with the lid on for about 40 minutes, or until the rice and carrots are tender; check after30 minutes.
5. Once the kale has wilted, cook for a few more minutes before adding the meatballs, salt, and pepper. If desired, add extra Parmesan cheese as a garnish.

   Nutritional Information: Calories: 229; Carbs: 8.3g; Fat: 7.7g; Protein: 32.2g

Chicken Noodle Soup with Bok Choy

Prep time: 10 minutes
Cooking time: 10-15 minutes
Servings: 4

Ingredients:

- 8 cups low-fodmap chicken or vegetable stock
- 1 heaping tablespoon grated ginger
- 4 kaffir lime leaves
- 1-pound boneless, skinless chicken breasts, very thinly sliced
- 8 oz gluten-free rice vermicelli, broken into 2-inch pieces
- 3 bunches of baby bok choy, leaves separated, rinsed & drained
- 1/2 cup bean sprouts
- 2 tsp gluten-free soy sauce

Instructions:

1. In a large, heavy-bottomed saucepan, bring the stock, ginger, and lime leaves to a boil. For five minutes, fry the chicken over low heat.
2. Simmer the rice noodles, bok choy, and bean sprouts for 5 minutes, or until they are tender.
   Before serving, take the lime leaves out and combine them with the soy sauce.
   Nutritional Information: Calories: 317; Carbs: 16g; Fat: 5.7g; Protein:7g

Curried Potato and Parsnip Soup

Prep time: 10 minutes
Cooking time: 30 minutes
Servings: 4

Ingredients:

- 1 tbsp canola oil
- 2 parsnips, peeled & cut into 3/4-inch pieces
- 4 potatoes, peeled & cut into 3/4-inch pieces
- 6 1/2 cups low-fodmap chicken or vegetable stock
- 1 tsp gluten-free curry powder, or to taste
- 1 cup low-fat milk, lactose-free milk, or suitable plant-based milk
- Salt & freshly ground black pepper
- Chopped flat-leaf parsley to garnish

Instructions:

1. Heat the canola oil in a large heavy-bottomed pot over medium heat.
2. Cook the potatoes and parsnips for 3 to 5 minutes, stirring often, until they are lightly browned.
3. Boil the stock for three minutes, then turn off the heat. When the vegetables are soft, reduce the heat to low and simmer for 15 to 20 minutes, stirring periodically.
4. Take the food off the heat and let it cool for 10 minutes. Make a smooth mixture using an immersion blender.
5. Combine the milk and curry powder in a blender, season with salt and pepper to taste. Reheat slowly without boiling. Garnish with a little sprinkle of parsley before serving.

Nutritional Information: Calories: 218; Carbs: 36g; Fat: 7g; Protein: 8g

Roasted Squash and Chestnut Soup

Prep time: 15 minutes
Cooking time: 60 minutes
Servings: 4

Ingredients:

- 2 pounds peeled, seeded, & cubed kabocha or other suitable winter squash
- 2 tbsp olive oil
- 2 cups unsweetened chestnut puree
- 8 cups low-fodmap chicken or vegetable stock
- 2 tsp ground ginger
- 1 cup low-fodmap milk, warmed
- Salt & freshly ground black pepper

Instructions:

1. Set the oven's temperature to 350°F.
2. Spread the squash out on a baking sheet and drizzle with olive oil. Bake for 30 to 40 minutes, turning often, until golden and well cooked.
3. Put the squash in a big stockpot or saucepan. Bring to a boil the stock, chestnut purée, and ginger.
4. Once the heat is reduced to medium-low, simmer the squash for 15 to 20 minutes, stirring periodically, or until it is tender. Give yourself ten minutes to cool down.
5. Using an immersion blender, puree the soup until it is absolutely smooth.
6. To taste, add salt and pepper. Serve with an extra milk swish on top (if preferred).
Nutritional Information: Calories: 437; Carbs: 31g; Fat: 12g; Protein: 21g

Creamy Seafood Soup

Prep time: 15 minutes
Cooking time: 30 minutes
Servings: 6

Ingredients:

- 3 tbsp salted butter
- 2 large carrots, diced
- 1/2 cup of long-grain white rice
- 5 cups chicken stock
- 4 tsp fish sauce
- 1/2 cup tomato puree
- 1/2 fennel bulb, finely chopped
- 1/2 cup white wine (optional)
- 1-pound raw medium shrimp, peeled & deveined
- 2 large or 5 small squid bodies, cleaned & sliced
- 5 oz boneless, skinless, firm fish fillets, cut into cubes
- 6 cooked jumbo shrimp
- 1 cup low-fodmap milk
- Salt & freshly ground black pepper to taste
- Extra virgin olive oil, to garnish (optional)

Instructions:

1. Melt the butter in a large, heavy-bottomed pot over medium heat.
2. After adding the rice and carrots, cook for 5 minutes while frequently stirring. Stock, fish sauce, tomato puree, fennel, and wine are combined in a bowl (if using).
3. Bring to a boil, reduce heat to low, and simmer for an additional 20 minutes, or until the rice is cooked through.
4. Give a cooling time of 10 minutes. Make a smooth mixture using an immersion blender.
5. Put the pan back on the flame and boil the soup for five minutes. Fish, squid, and shrimp should all be added raw to

the saucepan and cooked for 4 to 5 minutes, or until just done.

6. Once the milk and jumbo shrimp are fully heated and combined, add them.

7. Add olive oil, if desired, and season with salt and pepper to taste before serving.

Nutritional Information: Calories: 241; Carbs: 4g; Fat: 18g; Protein: 17g

Potato and Corn Chowder

Prep time: 15 minutes
Cooking time: 20-25 minutes
Servings: 6

Ingredients:

- 8 ounces lean bacon slices, diced (optional)
- Nonstick cooking spray
- 3 large potatoes, peeled (if desired) & diced
- 8 cups chicken or vegetable stock
- 1 (14.7-oz) can no-salt-add, gluten-free cream-style corn
- 1 tsp ground mustard
- 1 tsp fresh thyme leaves
- 1 tbsp roughly chopped flat-leaf parsley
- Salt & freshly ground black pepper to taste

Instructions:

1. In a large heavy-bottomed saucepan over medium heat, sauté bacon, if using, until crisp, turning periodically.
2. Transfer to a plate that has been covered with paper towels to drain. Apply cooking spray to the same saucepan, add the potatoes, and cook, often tossing, over medium heat.
3. Boil the stock for three minutes, then turn off the heat. After stirring the potatoes occasionally for 15 minutes, lower the heat to a low setting.
4. Utilizing an immersion blender, combine until smooth. After adding the corn, mustard, thyme, parsley, and saved bacon, season it with salt and pepper.
5. After a little warming without boiling, serve.
Nutritional Information: Calories: 284; Carbs: 46g; Fat: 7.3g; Protein: 12g

Lamb Shank and Vegetable Soup

Prep time: 15 minutes
Cooking time: 1 hour & 15 minutes
Servings: 4
Ingredients:

- 3 tbsp olive oil
- 1 tbsp garlic-infused olive oil
- 2 lamb shanks
- 1 1/2 pounds kabocha or other suitable winter squash, peeled, seeded, & cut into 3/4 inch pieces
- 3 large carrots, cut into 1/3-inch pieces
- 3 celery stalks, cut into 1/3-inch slices
- 6 1/2 cups beef stock
- 2/3 cup long-grain white rice

Instructions:

1. Heat the olive oil and garlic-infused oil over medium heat in a large heavy-bottomed pot.
2. Sear the lamb shanks for 2 to 3 minutes on each side before turning, cooking for a total of 5 to10 minutes, or until they are only barely browned on both sides.
3. Take the shanks out of the skillet and arrange them on a serving dish. Cook the squash, carrots, and celery for 2 to 3 minutes, until they are softly browned in the remaining oil and meat juices.
4. Put the pan back over medium-high heat and add the shanks. After stirring frequently for 50 to 60 minutes after bringing the liquid and rice to a boil, reduce the heat to low.
5. After removing the lamb shanks from the bones, slice or shred the meat into substantial chunks. Fat and bones need to be thrown away.
6. Add the lamb back to the pan and give it a good swirl, breaking up the bits of squash as you go.

7. Before serving, season with salt and pepper to taste.

   Nutritional Information: Calories: 381; Carbs: 14g; Fat: 18g; Protein: 37g

Lemon Chicken and Rice Soup

Prep time: 15 minutes
Cooking time: 50-55 minutes Servings: 6-8
Ingredients:

- 8 cups water
- 1 tbsp olive oil
- 2 pounds boneless skinless chicken thighs, visible fat removed, sliced
- Grated zest & juice of 2 lemons
- 1 tbsp superfine sugar
- 1 cup white rice
- 3 stalks of celery, finely sliced
- 1 tbsp chopped flat-leaf parsley
- Salt & freshly ground black pepper to taste

Instructions:

1. Heat the oil over medium-high heat in a large, heavy-bottomed pan. Cook the chicken, often flipping it, until golden brown on all sides.

2. Bring to a boil 8 cups of water. Set to low heat, cover, and simmer with the lemon juice and zest for 20 to 30 minutes (including the excess liquid).

3. After adding the rice to the pan, cook for 10 minutes.

4. After adding the celery, continue cooking for an additional 5 minutes, or until the rice is tender. Add the parsley and season to taste, then serve immediately.

   Nutritional Information: Calories: 315; Carbs: 38g; Fat: 8g; Protein: 19g

Potato and Parsnip Soup

Prep time: 15 minutes
Cooking time: 30-35 minutes
Servings: 4

Ingredients:

- 1 tbsp canola oil
- 1 stalk celery, very thinly sliced
- 6 parsnips, peeled & finely diced
- 2 potatoes, peeled & finely diced
- 3 cups low-fodmap vegetable stock
- 1/2 cup low-fat milk, lactose-free milk, or suitable plant-based milk
- 1/3 cup crumbled feta
- Salt & freshly ground black pepper
- 2 tbsp chopped chives

Instructions:

1. Heat the oil in a medium saucepan over medium heat. Cook the celery for 5 to 6 minutes, or until it is tender and well browned.
2. Add the potatoes and parsnips and cook for 1 to 2 minutes, stirring regularly. Allow it to boil, then reduce the heat to low, cover it, and simmer for 15 to 20 minutes, or until the vegetables are tender.
3. Turn off the heat, and then set the pot aside to cool for ten minutes. Working in batches, if necessary, combine the vegetables and stock in a food processor.
4. Until well-combined, add the milk and feta cheese. Re-add the soup to the pan and cook over medium heat, stirring often, until it just begins to boil.
5. After taking it off the heat, season with salt and pepper. Four dishes should contain the soup, with the chives diced on top.

Nutritional Information: Calories: 278; Carbs: 29g; Fat: 8g; Protein: 8g

Pork Ragout

Prep time: 15 minutes
Cooking time: 2 hours
Servings: 8

Ingredients:

- 3 tbsp garlic-infused canola oil
- 3-to 4-pound bone-in pork leg or center-cut pork loin, trimmed of fat
- 2 carrots, peeled & diced
- 2 stalks of celery, diced
- 2 bay leaves
- 2 tbsp chopped sage leaves
- 2 cups low-fodmap chicken stock
- 1 (28-oz) can of tomato puree
- 4 Yukon Gold potatoes, diced
- Salt & freshly ground black pepper
- Polenta, rice, gluten-free pasta, or mashed potatoes

Instructions:

1. Heat 2 tablespoons of the oil in a large flameproof casserole over medium-high heat.
2. Cook the pork for 2 to 3 minutes on each side, or until browned. Put the pork on a dish after removing it from the pan.
3. Simmer the carrots, celery, bay leaves, and sage in the remaining oil in the same saucepan for5 minutes, or until the vegetables are tender, stirring often.
4. In a large mixing bowl, combine the meat, potatoes, tomato puree, and stock. Bring to a boil, then reduce the heat to a low setting and cover.
5. Continue to simmer for 1 1/2 hours or until the pork is done, basting and turning the pig often.6. Remove, then turn the

heat up to medium-high to bring the sauce to a boil. 20 minutes of simmering should be plenty to thicken the sauce. 6.Cut the meat into large bits and remove it from the bone before adding it to the sauce. Serve.

Nutritional Information: Calories: 466; Carbs: 18g; Fat: 16g; Protein: 38g

Orange Chicken Soup

Prep time: 15 minutes
Cooking time: 15-20 minutes
Servings: 16
Ingredients:

- 4 quarts of chicken broth
- 1 /4 cup uncooked white or brown rice
- 1-pound carrots, peeled and coarsely chopped
- 1 small butternut or acorn squash, peeled & coarsely chopped
- 2 medium yams/sweet potatoes, peeled & coarsely chopped
- 1 tsp lemon juice

Instructions:

1. Place the rice and chicken stock in a big saucepan and heat to a boil. Include the yams, squash, and carrots.
2. Cook the veggies over low heat for 10 to 15 minutes, stirring periodically, until they are mushy.
3. Using an immersion blender, puree the soup until it is smooth. the pot with the blended soup.
   Stir thoroughly, then plate.
   Nutritional Information: Calories: 333; Carbs: 22g; Fat: 9g; Protein: 21g

Creamy Broccoli Soup

Prep time: 10 minutes + chilling time
Cooking time: 0 minutes
Servings: 4

Ingredients:

- 1 1/2 cups raw cashews, soaked for 2 hours
- 2 cups chopped broccoli
- 2 cups water
- 1 /8 tsp each salt & black pepper, or to taste
- 1 /4 tsp each powdered sage & dried thyme

Instructions:

1. After soaking the raw cashews for at least two hours, drain and rinse them.
2. Blend the cashews, broccoli, water, and optional spices until completely smooth. After mixing, refrigerate the soup in the fridge for approximately 30 minutes. Serve.

Nutritional Information: Calories: 287; Carbs: 18g; Fat: 8g; Protein: 13g

Curry Spinach Soup

Prep time: 10 minutes

Cooking time: 0 minutes

Servings: 2

Ingredients:

- 1 bunch of fresh spinach
- 1 /4 cup fresh dill
- 1 /2 of a red bell pepper
- 1 small ripe tomato
- 1/2 avocado, pitted & sliced
- 1 tbsp low-fodmap Nama Shoyu (raw organic soy sauce)
- 2 tsp lemon juice
- 1 tsp curry powder
- 1/2 cup of water
- 1 /2 diced red or orange bell pepper

Instructions:

1. Combine all the ingredients in a food processor or blender.
2. Once the mixture is smooth, serve.
   Nutritional Information: Calories: 256; Carbs: 32g; Fat: 8g; Protein:11g

Potato Leek Soup

Prep time: 10 minutes

Cooking time: 15 minutes

Servings: 4

Ingredients:

- 6 cups vegetable broth
- 5 russet potatoes, peeled & chopped
- 2 leeks, green parts only, thoroughly washed & chopped
- ½ tsp sea salt
- 1/8 tsp freshly ground black pepper

Instructions:

1. Stir the potatoes, leeks, salt, and pepper into the stock in a big saucepan over medium-high heat. The soup should boil.
2. Lower the heat to low and let the soup simmer for around 10 minutes, or until the potatoes and leeks are tender.
3. Purée the soup in a blender or food processor, if necessary, in stages, until it is smooth.
   Nutritional Information: Calories:234; Carbs: 55g; Fat: <1g; Protein: 5g

Quinoa Soup with Miso

Prep time: 10 minutes
Cooking time: 30-35 minutes
Servings: 8

Ingredients:

- 2 tbsp olive oil
- 2 carrots, sliced & cut in half moons
- 2 celery stalks, sliced
- 2 medium red potatoes, cut in quarter moons with skin
- 1 zucchini, cut in quarter moons
- 1 tsp salt
- 3 cups low-fodmap chicken stock
- 2 cups water
- 1 cup cooked quinoa
- 1 /2 tsp dry basil
- 1 /4 tsp dry oregano
- 3 tbsp white miso paste

Instructions:

1. Sauté the carrots and celery for 5 minutes in hot olive oil in a medium saucepan.
2. In a large basin, mix the potatoes, zucchini, salt, chicken stock, and water. After bringing everything to a boil, turn down the heat for 15 minutes.
3. In the meantime, make the quinoa as directed on the box.
4. In a medium saucepan, combine the cooked quinoa, basil, and oregano and heat for 5 minutes.
   Turn off the heat. The white miso paste should be well dissolved after being added.

Nutritional Information: Calories: 245; Carbs: 32g; Fat: 8g; Protein: 11g

Greens And Lemon Soup

Prep time: 10 minutes

Cooking time: 15 minutes

Servings: 4

Ingredients:

- 2 tbsp garlic oil
- 5 scallions, green parts only, chopped
- 5 cups stemmed, chopped Swiss chard
- 6 cups low-fodmap vegetable broth
- ½ tsp sea salt
- ¼ tsp freshly ground black pepper
- juice of 2 lemons

Instructions:

1. In a large saucepan, heat the garlic oil over medium-high heat until it shimmers. Add the chard and scallions. While stirring, cook for 3 minutes.
2. Add the broth along with the salt and pepper. 10 minutes of simmering with periodic stirring.

   Add the lemon juice, then serve.

   Nutritional Information: Calories:106; Carbs: 11g; Fat: 7g; Protein: 2g

Chicken Noodle Soup

Prep time: 10 minutes
Cooking time: 25-30 minutes
Servings: 4

Ingredients:

- 2 tbsp garlic oil
- 6 scallions, green parts only, chopped
- 3 carrots, chopped
- 1 red bell pepper, chopped
- 6 cups low-fodmap poultry broth
- ½ tsp sea salt
- 1/8 tsp freshly ground black pepper
- 4 oz gluten-free spaghetti, cooked according to Instructions: on the package
- 4 cups chopped cooked chicken

Instructions:

1. In a large saucepan, heat the garlic oil over medium-high heat until it shimmers. Add the bell pepper, carrots, and scallions. With occasional stirring, cook for 3 minutes.
2. Add the broth along with the salt and pepper. Make it boil. The spaghetti should be added at this point, and it should be cooked for 8 to 10 minutes while being stirred periodically. Good drainage
3. Add the chicken and cook for another 2 minutes. Serve.
   Nutritional Information: Calories: 441; Carbs: 24g; Fat: 35g; Protein: 52g

Vegetable Beef Soup

Prep time: 15 minutes
Cooking time: 15 minutes
Servings: 4
Ingredients:

- 1 pound of ground beef
- 7 cups low-fodmap poultry broth
- 6 scallions, green parts only, chopped
- 2 carrots, chopped
- 1 zucchini, chopped
- 1 red bell pepper, chopped
- 1 tsp dried thyme
- ½ tsp sea salt
- 1/8 tsp freshly ground black pepper

Instructions:

1. Brown the ground beef for approximately 5 minutes in a large saucepan over medium-high heat, breaking it up with the back of a spoon.
2. Include the broth, thyme, bell pepper, scallions, zucchini, carrots, and salt and pepper. Reduce the heat to medium after bringing the soup to a simmer.
3. Cook the vegetables until they are crisp-tender for about 7 minutes, stirring periodically. Add the cabbage and stir. three more minutes of cooking.
   Nutritional Information: Calories:279; Carbs: 11g; Fat: 7g; Protein: 40g

Nutty Summer Fruit Salad

Prep time: 10 minutes
Cooking time: 0 minutes Servings: 4-6

Ingredients:

- 5 tbsp brown sugar
- ¼ cup red wine vinegar
- ½ tsp mustard powder
- ½ tsp Himalayan salt
- 1 tbsp poppy seeds
- ½ cup sunflower oil
- 2 tsp. vegan mayonnaise
- 5-6 cups iceberg lettuce, chopped
- ¾ cup toasted pecans, chopped
- ¼ cup cardinal grapes, chopped
- 1 cup pineapple chunks
- ¼ cup fresh blueberries
- ½ cup fresh strawberries, sliced

Instructions:

1. Pulse the sugar and red wine vinegar in a food processor until the majority of the sugar grains have dissolved. Add the salt, poppy seeds, and mustard powder.
2. Add the oil and mayonnaise gradually when the food processor is nearing capacity. Place the sauce in a basin and refrigerate while assembling the salad.
3. Combine the lettuce, nuts, grapes, pineapple, blueberries, strawberries, and 4-6 tablespoons of dressing in a large bowl. Serve.
   Nutritional Information: Calories: 134; Carbs: 26g; Fat: 1g; Protein: 2g

Fried Tofu Puffs Spinach & Bell Pepper Salad

Prep time: 15 minutes

Cooking time: 0 minutes

Servings: 4

Ingredients:

- 1/4 cup gluten-free soy sauce
- 1/4 cup fresh lemon juice
- 1 tbsp + 1 tsp seasoned rice vinegar
- 1/4 cup packed light brown sugar
- 1/4 cup sesame oil
- 10 cups baby spinach leaves, rinsed & dried
- 1 1/2 cups snow pea shoots or bean sprouts
- 1 green bell pepper, seeded and sliced
- 14 oz fried tofu puffs, cut into cubes
- 1/3 cup pine nuts
- Salt & freshly ground black pepper to taste

Instructions:

1. In a small bowl, combine the soy sauce, lemon juice, vinegar, brown sugar, and sesame oil.
2. Combine the spinach, snow pea shoots, bell pepper, tofu, and pine nuts in a large mixing dish.3. Pour the dressing over the salad and give it a quick swirl. Serve after taste-testing and adding salt and pepper.

   Nutritional Information: Calories: 143; Carbs: 16g; Fat: 3.2g; Protein:11g

Peppered Beef and Citrus Salad

Prep time: 15 minutes + chilling time
Cooking time: 8 minutes
Servings: 1

Ingredients:

- 2 tsp olive oil
- 1-pound beef sirloin or top round steak
- 2 tsp garlic-infused olive oil
- 1 tbsp freshly ground black pepper, + more for serving
- 1/4 cup fresh lemon juice
- 1 tbsp light brown sugar
- Salt to taste
- 1 orange, peeled & cut into segments
- 1 head butter lettuce (Boston or Bibb), leaves separated
- 1 (8-oz) can of water chestnuts, drained and roughly chopped

Instructions:

1. Heat the olive oil in a frying pan over medium heat.
2. To cook the steak to your preferred doneness, cook it for 4 minutes on each side for medium rare. Before slicing the steak thinly, let it rest for 10 minutes.
3. In a medium bowl, combine the garlic-infused oil, pepper, lemon juice, brown sugar, and salt to taste.
4. Stir the meat into the marinade until it is well coated. 3 hours in the refrigerator under cover.5. Combine the meat, lettuce, water chestnuts, and any remaining marinade in a large mixing dish. Add a couple grinds of black pepper to the dish before serving.

Nutritional Information: Calories: 305; Carbs: 2g; Fat: 27g; Protein: 15g

Spiced Lamb Roasted Sweet Potato Salad

Prep time: 15 minutes
Cooking time: 36-40 minutes
Servings: 4
Ingredients:

- 4 small, sweet potatoes, peeled (if desired) & cut into 3⁄4-inch cubes
- 1 red bell pepper, seeded & cut into quarters
- Olive oil, as needed
- 1 tbsp ground cumin
- 2 tsp ground coriander
- ½ tsp ground cardamom
- 2 tsp ground turmeric
- ½ tsp ground sumac
- 1-pound lean lamb steak, cut into thin strips
- 8 oz baby spinach leaves (8 cups), rinsed and dried

Instructions:

1. Set the oven's temperature to 350°F. On a large baking sheet, olive oil should be brushed over the bell pepper and sweet potato.
2. Cook the veggies for 30 minutes, or until they are tender and browned. Await cooling Once the bell pepper has cooled enough to handle, peel off the skin.
3. In a medium frying pan, warm some olive oil over low heat. Add the sumac, cumin, coriander, cardamom, and heat for one minute or until fragrant.
4. Add the lamb and stir to evenly distribute the spice mixture. Cook, stirring regularly, for 3 to 5 minutes, or until gently browned. Cut the heat off.
5. Combine the spinach, sweet potato, and bell pepper in a large mixing bowl. Add a final drizzle of olive oil before serving the lamb with any pan juices.

Nutritional Information: Calories: 287; Carbs: 26g; Fat: 12g; Protein: 7g

DESSERTS

Chocolate-Drizzled Raspberry Muffins

Prep time: 15 minutes
Cooking time: 20 minutes Servings: 12 muffins
Ingredients:

- 6 tbsp butter, cubed
- 2 ½ cups gluten-free self-rising flour
- ½ cup dark chocolate, roughly chopped
- 1 cup raspberries
- 1 cup almond milk
- 1 tsp chia seeds, soaked in 2 tbsp water
- Icing sugar for dusting

Instructions:

1. Butter a muffin tray liberally and preheat the oven to 375°F with a wire rack in the center.
2. Using your hands, mash the butter and flour in a large basin until the mixture resembles gritty sand.
3. Include the chia seeds, chocolate, raspberries, and almond milk. Fold until all ingredients are barely mixed.
4. Evenly distribute the mixture into the muffin tray that has been preheated, and bake for 15-20minutes, or until the tops are brown.
5. Before moving the muffins to a cooling rack, let them cool in the pan for 5 minutes. When somewhat cooled, sprinkle with icing sugar and serve warm.
   Nutritional Information: Calories: 233; Carbs: 39g; Fat: 8g; Protein: 5g

Rich Walnut Brownies

Prep time: 10 minutes

Cooking time: 10 minutes Servings: 24 brownies

Ingredients:

- 1/8 tsp Himalayan salt
- 1 cup pure cocoa powder
- 2 ½ cups icing sugar
- 3 egg whites (more if needed)
- 1 cup toasted walnuts, roughly chopped
- 2 tsp pure vanilla essence

Instructions:

1. Place a wire rack in the center of the oven and line a baking pan with greaseproof paper. Setthe oven to preheat to 350°F.
2. In a large basin, combine the icing sugar, cocoa powder, and salt. Using a wooden spoon, gently fold the egg whites until a thick dough forms. Add the nuts and vanilla extract by blending them.
3. Place batter balls on the preheated baking sheet using an ice cream scoop. Bake the sheet for10 minutes, or until the tops of the brownies begin to crack.
4. Before serving, let the brownies cool completely on the pan.
   Nutritional Information: Calories: 160; Carbs: 23g; Fat: 7g; Protein: 2g

Amaretti

Prep time: 15 minutes
Cooking time: 18-25 minutes Servings: 20-25 biscuits

Ingredients:

- 1 cup almond flour, preferably finely ground
- 3/4 cup confectioners' sugar
- 1 tbsp + 1 tsp cornstarch
- 2 large egg whites
- 1/3 cup superfine sugar
- 1 tsp almond extract

Instructions:

1. Line two baking pans with parchment paper and preheat the oven to 350°F.
2. In a medium basin, combine the cornstarch, confectioners' sugar, and almond flour.
3. Using an electric hand mixer, whisk the egg whites in a clean, medium mixing bowl until soft peaks form.
4. After adding the superfine sugar, whisk the mixture until glossy, firm peaks form. Almond extract should be added and thoroughly mixed.
5. Gently incorporate the almond flour mixture into the batter using a large metal spoon until just mixed. Place tablespoon-sized mounds of batter on the baking sheets, giving them room to spread.

   Until golden brown, bake for 18 to 25 minutes. Let it cool before serving.

   Nutritional Information: Calories: 241; Carbs: 23g; Fat: 10g; Protein: 8g

Banana Friands

Prep time: 15 minutes

Cooking time: 20 minutes Servings: 12 friands

Ingredients:

- 9 tbsp unsalted butter, cut into cubes
- 1/4 cup confectioners' sugar, + more for dusting
- 1/4 cup cornstarch
- 1/4 cup superfine white rice flour
- 1 1/4 cups almond flour
- 5 large egg whites, lightly beaten
- 1 tbsp + 1 tsp fresh lemon juice
- 1 tsp vanilla extract
- 1 small ripe banana, peeled & roughly chopped

Instructions:

1. Set the oven to 350°F and use cooking spray to gently grease a 12-cup muffin pan.
2. Melt the butter in a small skillet over low heat, then cook for a further 3 to 4 minutes, or until brown flecks appear. Take it out of the equation.
3. In a large mixing basin, sift the rice flour, cornstarch, and confectioners' sugar three times.
4. Stir in the almond flour after which, using a large metal spoon, whisk together the egg whites, lemon juice, vanilla, and melted butter. Mix thoroughly after adding the pieces of banana.
5. Fill each cup two-thirds full with batter; bake for 12 to 15 minutes, or until firm and lightly browned.
6. Allow to cool in the pan for five minutes before transferring to a wire rack to finish cooling.

   Dust with confectioners' sugar just before serving.

   Nutritional Information: Calories: 299; Carbs: 28g Fat: 13g; Protein: 11g

Chocolate & Espresso Power Balls

Prep time: 10 minutes + chilling time
Cooking time: 0 minutes Servings: 12 balls
Ingredients:

- ¼ cup chocolate-covered espresso beans, crushed
- 2 tsp instant powdered espresso
- 4 tsp Dutch-processed cocoa
- 1/3 cup rice syrup
- 1/8 tsp vanilla extract
- 1 cup old-fashioned oats
- ½ cup creamy peanut butter

Instructions:

1. In a large bowl, add all the ingredients—save for the crushed chocolate-dipped espresso beans—and stir well to blend.
2. After incorporating the espresso beans, refrigerate for 30 minutes in the fridge. Make 1-inchdiameter bite-sized balls out of the mixture. 12 balls should be made from the mixture.
3. Keep in the freezer for up to a month or the refrigerator for a week.
   Nutritional Information: Calories 174; Fat 8g; Carbs 22g; Protein 6g

Cantaloupe Lime Popsicles

Prep time: 10 minutes + freezing time
Cooking time: 12 minutes
Servings: 6

Ingredients:

- 20 oz ripe orange cantaloupe, cut into chunks
- 4 tsp freshly squeezed lime juice
- ¾ cup water
- ⅓ cup sugar

Instructions:

1. In a small saucepan, combine the water and sugar. Heat the mixture gently while constantly stirring until the sugar dissolves. Turn off the heat and let the food cool fully.
2. In a blender, combine all the ingredients, including the sugar water, and mix until completely smooth. Fill ice pop molds with the mixture and freeze until firm.
   Nutritional Information: Calories 62; Carbs 16g; Fat 1g; Protein 1g

White Chocolate & Cranberry Energy Balls

Prep time: 10 minutes + chilling time
Cooking time: 0 minutes Servings: 12 balls
Ingredients:

- 1/3 cup maple syrup or rice syrup
- ½ cup dried cranberries, coarsely chopped
- 2/3 cup white chocolate chips
- ½ cup natural peanut butter
- 1 cup old-fashioned oats
- 1/8 tsp vanilla extract

Instructions:

1. In a large bowl, add all the ingredients and stir well to blend. For 30 minutes, chill in the refrigerator.
2. Form the mixture into bite-sized balls with a diameter of approximately 1 inch. 12 balls should be made from the mixture. Keep in the freezer for up to a month or the refrigerator for a week.
   Nutritional Information: Calories 243; Carbs 37g; Fat 9g; Protein 6g

Berry Friands

Prep time: 15 minutes
Cooking time: 19-20 minutes Servings: 12 friands
Ingredients:

- Nonstick cooking spray
- 9 tbsp unsalted butter, cut into cubes
- 1 1/2 cup confectioners' sugar, + more for dusting
- 1/4 cup cornstarch
- 1/4 cup superfine white rice flour
- 1 1/4 cup almond flour
- 5 large egg whites, lightly beaten
- 1 tbsp + 1 tsp fresh lemon juice
- 2 tsp vanilla extract
- 1 cup blueberries or raspberries

Instructions:

1. Set the oven to 350°F and use cooking spray to gently grease a 12-cup muffin pan.
2. Melt the butter in a small skillet over low heat, then cook for a further 3 to 4 minutes, or until brown flecks appear. Take it out of the equation.
3. In a large mixing bowl, sift the rice flour, cornstarch, and confectioners' sugar three times.
4. Stir in the almond flour, after which, using a large metal spoon, whisk together the egg whites, lemon juice, vanilla, and melted butter.
5. Fill each cup with the batter until it is two-thirds full. Gently push 4 berries into the center of each friand.
6. Bake for 12 to 15 minutes, or until firm and lightly golden. Cool in the pan for five minutes before transferring to a wire rack to finish cooling. dust with confectioners' sugar just before serving.
Nutritional Information: Calories: 237; Carbs: 25g; Fat: 9g; Protein: 11g

Chocolate Truffles

Prep time: 15 minutes + chilling time
Cooking time: 0 minutes Servings: 25 truffles
Ingredients:

- 7 oz gluten-free vanilla cookies, finely crushed
- 1/3 cup unsweetened cocoa powder
- 1/3 cup sweetened condensed milk
- 2 tbsp rum or brandy (optional)
- 1 1/2 cup gluten-free chocolate sprinkles

Instructions:

1. Combine the cocoa and cookie crumbs in a medium mixing bowl. With your hands, combine the condensed milk and rum (if using) until a firm dough forms.
2. Add the chocolate sprinkles to a small plate. Make balls out of teaspoons of the truffle mixture using your hands.
3. Add the chocolate sprinkles to the coat. Refrigerate the mixture until it becomes firm.
   Nutritional Information: Calories: 311; Carbs: 16g; Fat: 7.1g; Protein: 44g

Banana Fritters with Fresh Pineapple

Prep time: 15 minutes

Cooking time: 6-8 minutes

Servings: 2

Ingredients:

- 1 cup dried gluten-free, soy-free bread crumbs
- 1/3 cup packed light brown sugar
- 1 tbsp ground cinnamon
- 2 large eggs
- ½ tsp confectioners' sugar
- 4 small bananas, peeled & halved lengthwise
- 2 tbsp unsalted butter
- Gluten-free, lactose-free vanilla ice cream for serving
- 1/2 small pineapple, peeled, cored, & finely chopped
- Pulp of 2 passion fruits (optional)

Instructions:

1. Set the oven to 300 Fahrenheit. On a large dish, mix the cinnamon, brown sugar, and breadcrumbs.
2. In a small basin, lightly whisk the eggs with the confectioners' sugar. After dipping the banana halves into the egg mixture, cover them well with bread crumbs.
3. In a large nonstick frying pan over medium-low heat, melt 1 tablespoon of the butter. Cook the first half of the banana slices for 3 to 4 minutes on each side, or until they are golden brown.
4. Move to a baking pan, then reheat in the oven. Cook the remaining banana halves in the same manner with the remaining 1 tablespoon of butter after melting it.
5. Distribute four plates with two banana halves each. Add ice cream, pineapple, and passionfruit pulp as garnishes (if desired). Serve right away.

Nutritional Information: Calories: 274; Carbs: 6g; Fat: 18g; Protein: 23g

Shortbread Fingers

Prep time: 20 minutes

Cooking time: 35 minutes Servings: 36 shortbread fingers

Ingredients:

- 1 cup confectioners' sugar
- 1 tbsp + 2 tsp vanilla sugar, + more for sprinkling
- 2 cups cornstarch, + more for kneading
- 1 cup soy flour
- 1/2 cup superfine white rice flour
- 2 tsp xanthan gum or guar gum
- 1 cup unsalted butter, cut into cubes at room temperature

Instructions:

1. Combine the confectioners' sugar, vanilla sugar, cornstarch, soy flour, rice flour, and xanthan gum in a food processor or blender and pulse until well combined.
2. Add the butter and process for an additional 3 to 5 minutes to create a dough. Dust your worksurface lightly with cornstarch.
3. Spread the dough out on the work area and knead it softly until it comes together. The dough should be rolled out between two sheets of parchment paper to a thickness of 12 inches.
4. Arrange in 2 x 34-inch rectangles on prepared baking sheets, leaving some space for spreading. Add more vanilla sugar on top.
5. Set the oven to 200°F, then bake the food for 20 to 25 minutes, or until golden brown. Bake the food for a further 10 minutes at 200°F until golden brown.
6. Cool on the sheets for 10 to 12 minutes before moving to a wire rack to finish cooling.

Nutritional Information: Calories: 122; Carbs:13g; Fat: 13g; Protein: 16g

Bread Pudding with Blueberries

Prep time: 10 minutes
Cooking time: 40 minutes
Servings: 2
Ingredients:

- 1 extra-large egg
- 2/3 cup unsweetened almond milk
- 1 tbsp maple syrup
- ¼ tsp vanilla extract
- 4 slices of gluten-free bread
- ½ cup blueberries
- A dash of ground cinnamon

Instructions:

1. Set the oven to 375 degrees.
2. In a bowl, thoroughly blend the eggs, almond milk, and maple syrup. Put the vanilla extract there.
3. Slice the bread into little pieces after removing the crusts. In a greased baking dish, add the bread pieces and the egg mixture.
4. Add some blueberries on top and a splash of cinnamon. Bake for 40 minutes, or until the top is golden and puffy and the egg mixture has set.
   Nutritional Information: Calories 268; Carbs 44.9g; Fat 6.5g; Protein 7.8g

Millet Chocolate Pudding

Prep time: 10 minutes + chilling time
Cooking time: 0 minutes
Servings: 4

Ingredients:

- 1 lb. cooked millet
- 2 cups unsweetened almond milk
- ½ medium banana
- ¼ cup cocoa powder
- 2 tbsp maple syrup

Instructions:

1. Add all the ingredients to a blender, and pulse until everything is well combined.
2. Place the dishes with the chocolate mixture in the refrigerator to set for a few minutes before serving.
   Nutritional Information: Calories 260; Carbs 45.9g; Fat 5.8g; Protein 8.9g

Chocolate English Custard

Prep time: 10 minutes + chilling time
Cooking time: 10 minutes
Servings: 2
Ingredients:

- 1 ½ tbsp tapioca starch
- 1 egg
- 1 tbsp pure maple syrup
- ¾ cup almond milk
- 1 tbsp water
- 1 ½ tbsp cocoa powder

Instructions:

1. Place all the ingredients in a pot and whisk to ensure that there are no lumps.
2. Place the pot on the burner and, while continually stirring, bring to a boil over low heat. Once the mixture has thickened, turn the heat off.
3. Transfer to ramekins and chill for three hours before serving.
   Nutritional Information: Calories 170; Carbs 24.6g; Fat 6.5g; Protein 5.8g

Vanilla Maple Chia Pudding

Prep time: 10 minutes + chilling time

Cooking time: 0 minutes

Servings: 1

Ingredients:

- 3 tbsp chia seeds
- 1 cup coconut milk
- ½ tsp vanilla extract
- 1 tbsp maple syrup

Instructions:

1. In a bowl, add all the ingredients and toss to thoroughly blend.
2. Put in the refrigerator and let it sit for the night.
   Nutritional Information: Calories 280; Carbs 31.7g; Fat 12.6g; Protein 10.2g

Dark Chocolate Gelato

Prep time: 10 minutes + freezing time
Cooking time: 10 minutes Servings: 8-10
Ingredients:

- 2 ¼ cups coconut milk
- ¾ cup lactose-free heavy cream
- 2 tbsp arrowroot starch
- ½ cup cocoa powder
- 4 oz dark chocolate
- ¾ cup sugar

Instructions:

1. In a saucepan, combine half of the coconut milk, cream, arrowroot, cocoa powder, and dark chocolate. Include the sugar.
2. Start the burner, then cook the mixture until it thickens. Put the remaining milk in when the heat is turned off. combine well after mixing.
3. Put the mixture in a container with a lid and refrigerate for eight hours, stirring the mixture every hour to get the creamy gelato texture.
   Nutritional Information: Calories 145; Carbs 11g; Fat 11.4g; Protein 2.5g

Banana Cake

Prep time: 15 minutes
Cooking time: 45 minutes
Servings: 8

Ingredients:

- 4 oz softened butter
- 3 eggs
- 2 cups gluten-free flour
- 2 tsp baking powder
- 1 tsp cinnamon
- ½ cup Greek yogurt
- 1 cup mashed banana
- ¼ cup brown sugar

Instructions:

1. Preheat the oven to 350 degrees Fahrenheit and butter a baking pan.
2. Combine the butter and sugar in a bowl and combine with an electric mixer until the mixture is frothy and light in color. While stirring, gradually add the eggs.
3. Add the yogurt and banana to the butter mixture after sifting in the flour, baking powder, and cinnamon. Stir well to mix.
4. Pour the mixture into the baking dish and bake for 45 minutes, or until a toothpick inserted in the center of the mixture comes out clean. Before removing it from the baking dish, let it cool.

Nutritional Information: Calories 231; Carbs 18.6g; Fat 16.1g; Protein 5.1g

Butter Tarts

Prep time: 20 minutes

Cooking time: 30 minutes Servings: 24 tarts

Ingredients:

- 1 ½ cups gluten-free flour
- ¼ cup butter
- ¼ cup lard
- 1 egg yolk
- 1 tsp vinegar
- Iced water, as needed
- 1 egg
- 2 tbsp butter, room temperature
- 1 tsp vanilla
- 1 tsp vinegar
- ¼ tsp salt
- ¾ cup brown sugar

Instructions:

1. Set the oven to 350 degrees Fahrenheit and butter the tart pan.
2. To make the tart crust, stir the gluten-free flour into the butter and lard mixture. Continue doing this until a coarse meal forms.
3. Stir the egg yolk, vinegar, and a little bit of cold water in a bowl until the mixture is about 12 cups full.
4. Using your hands, gradually incorporate the ingredients into the crust to form a pastry dough. The dough should be pressed into tart pans and chilled for two hours to solidify.
5. In the meantime, mix together the sugar, butter, egg, vanilla, and vinegar. Add the salt and stir.
   combine well after mixing.
6. Pipe the tart filling into the prepared dough, then bake for 30 minutes in a 450°F preheated oven.
7. Allow it to cool before taking it out of the tart mold.

Nutritional Information: Calories 86; Carbs 8.4g; Fat 5.7g; Protein 0.6g.

Lime Cake

Prep time: 15 minutes
Cooking time: 45 minutes
Servings: 8

Ingredients:

- 2 ½ cups gluten-free flour
- 1 tbsp baking powder
- 1 tsp xanthan gum
- 4 large eggs
- 1 cup canola oil
- 1 cup coconut milk
- 1 tsp vanilla extract
- 1 tsp lime extract
- 2 cups sugar
- ½ tsp salt
- 1 tbsp lime zest
- 3 tbsp freshly squeezed lime juice

Instructions:

1. Grease a cake pan with shortening or oil and preheat the oven to 350°F.
2. In a bowl, combine the flour, baking powder, and xanthan gum. To aerate the dry ingredients, sift them through a sieve.
3. In a separate dish, combine the eggs, canola oil, coconut milk, lime juice, lime zest, sugar, salt, and lime essence. Beat the mixture until it becomes smooth, and the sugar has dissolved.
4. Gently fold the dry ingredients in, then stir to break up any lumps.
5. Transfer the batter to the prepared pan. To get rid of extra air in the batter, tap the pan's bottom. 45 minutes of baking should be done in the oven. Serve.

Nutritional Information: Calories 422; Carbs 35.2g; Fat 30.7g; Protein 3.1g

Berry Crumb Cake

Prep time: 20 minutes

Cooking time: 50 minutes Servings: 8 slices

Ingredients:

- 2 cups gluten-free flour
- 1 tsp baking powder
- ¾ cup butter, cold
- ¾ cup coconut milk
- 1 tbsp lemon juice
- 2 eggs
- 1 cup strawberries and blueberries
- 1 cup sugar

Instructions:

1. Lightly oil an 8x8 square pan and preheat the oven to 350°F.
2. Combine the sugar, baking powder, and sugar in a bowl.
3. Gradually incorporate the butter into the flour mixture. Achieve a crumb-like texture using a pastry blender; set aside half of the mixture for the topping.
4. Add the coconut milk and lemon juice to another bowl. Observe it for five minutes.
5. Combine the eggs, milk, and half of the flour mixture well. The berries are folded in.
6. Spoon the prepared mixture into the pan, then cover with the saved crumbs. Before slicing, let the cake cool after 50 minutes in the oven.

   Nutritional Information: Calories 171; Carbs 13.6g; Fat 12.7g; Protein 1.9g

Chocolate Chunks Cookies

Prep time: 10 minutes + chilling time
Cooking time: 15 minutes Servings: 14 cookies
Ingredients:
- 2 1/3 cup gluten-free flour
- 1 tsp baking soda
- 1 cup unsalted butter, room temperature
- 1 cup light brown sugar
- 2 tsp vanilla extract
- 2 large eggs
- 12 oz dark chocolates, chopped
- 1 1/3 cups toasted pecan halves, chopped
- 1 tsp salt

Instructions:
1. Combine the flour, baking soda, and salt in a bowl. To aerate, sift the flour mixture. Place aside.
2. Add the sugar and vanilla essence to a bowl with the butter. The mixture will brighten after 3 minutes of beating. One by one, include the eggs.
3. Add the dry ingredients and beat until there are just a few streaks of flour left.
4. Thoroughly mix the dark chocolates and pecans before adding them. For at least four hours, cover and refrigerate the bowl.
5. Set the oven to 375 degrees. Use parchment paper to cover a baking sheet. In the highest thirds of the oven, place the rack.
6. Make tiny balls out of the dough and put them on the baking sheet. Bake for 15 minutes, or until they are just beginning to turn light brown. Serve.
Nutritional Information: Calories 378; Carbs 32.2g; Fat 26.7g; Protein 4.1g

PB Oatmeal Chocolate Chip Cookies

Prep time: 10 minutes
Cooking time: 15 minutes
Servings: 4

Ingredients:

- 1 cup gluten-free flour
- ½ tsp xanthan gum
- 1 tsp baking soda
- 8 tbsp unsalted butter, cold & cubed
- ½ cup natural creamy peanut butter
- 2/3 cup sugar
- 1 tsp pure vanilla extract
- 1 large egg
- ¾ cup gluten-free quick oats
- 1 cup semi-sweet mini chocolate chips
- ¼ tsp salt

Instructions:

1. Line a baking sheet with parchment paper and preheat the oven to 350 degrees Fahrenheit.
2. In a small bowl, combine the salt, baking soda, xanthan gum, and gluten-free flour.
3. In a separate dish, combine the peanut butter, sugar, and vanilla essence with the butter. Add the eggs and continue beating until everything is properly blended.
4. Continue mixing after adding the dry ingredients gradually until all of them are combined.
5. Add the chocolate chip cookies and oats. Place a scoop of cookie dough on the baking sheet and bake for 12 minutes.
6. Before serving, remove from the cookie sheet and place on a cooling rack.

Nutritional Information: Calories 199; Carbs 25.5g; Fat 10.3g; Protein 4.2g

Baked Peanut Butter Protein Bars

Prep time: 15 minutes + chilling time
Cooking time: 1 minute Servings: 12 bars
Ingredients:
- 1 cup natural creamy peanut butter
- ¾ cup maple syrup
- 1 tsp vanilla bean paste
- 1 ½ cups gluten-free rolled oats
- 1 cup protein powder

Instructions:
1. Use parchment paper to line a baking sheet.
2. In a microwave-safe dish, warm the peanut butter and maple syrup for 30 seconds. After thoroughly stirring and adding the vanilla bean paste, re-heat for 30 seconds.
3. Add the protein powder and oats. Utilizing the back of the spoon, spread the mixture into the prepared pan. Cut into 12 bars after an hour in the refrigerator.

   Nutritional Information: Calories 271; Carbs 27.6g; Fat 14.9g; Protein 14g

Gluten-Free Lemon Cookies

Prep time: 10 minutes

Cooking time: 15 minutes Servings: 20 cookies

Ingredients:

- ¼ cup coconut milk
- ¼ cup fresh lemon juice
- ½ cup butter
- 1 egg
- 1 tsp vanilla extract
- Zest of one lemon
- 1 tsp baking soda
- 1 tsp baking powder
- 2 ½ cups gluten-free flour
- ½ cup fresh lemon juice
- 2 cups powdered sugar
- 1 cup sugar

Instructions:

1. Butter-grease a baking sheet and preheat the oven to 350°F. Place aside.
2. In a dish, mix the milk and lemon juice. Place aside.
3. With the aid of an electric mixer, cream the butter and sugar. Add the vanilla essence and the egg. Fold in the milk mixture after adding it to the butter mixture. Place aside.
4. In another basin, mix the flour, baking powder, and lemon zest. Fold after adding the dry ingredients to the wet ones.
5. Place a scoop of cookie dough on the baking pan. Use your fingers to press the dough; bake for 15 minutes. On a cooling rack, let the cookies cool.
6. In the meantime, make the frosting by combining sugar and lemon juice. The icing should be brushed over the cookies' tops.

Nutritional Information: Calories 110; Carbs 14.1g; Fat 5.9g; Protein 0.9g

Strawberry Frozen Yogurt

Prep time: 10 minutes

Cooking time: 0 minutes

Servings: 4

Ingredients:

- 1 cup strawberries, frozen
- 1 cup other fruit, chopped & frozen
- 1 cup plain thick lactose-free yogurt
- 1 tbsp caster sugar
- 1 tsp vanilla essence

Instructions:

1. Add all ingredients to a food processor and pulse just long enough to combine. Serve.

Nutritional Information: Calories 104; Carbs 14g; Fat 2g; Protein 5g

DRINKS & SMOOTHIES

Strawberry Basil Soda

Prep time: 10 minutes
Cooking time: 10 minutes
Servings: 1
Ingredients:

- ¼ cup brown sugar
- ¼ cup white sugar
- 1 cup water
- 1 cup strawberries
- ½ lemon, juiced
- 5 basil leaves
- Soda water, as needed

Instructions:

1. Heat enough water and sugar in a saucepan over medium heat until the mixture simmers.
2. After adding the strawberries to the saucepan, boil them for 5 minutes, stirring regularly to break up the berries.
3. After five minutes, turn off the heat and let the mixture cool to room temperature.
4. To make the syrup smooth, add the lemon juice and strawberry mixture to a blender.
5. Gently stir a cup of soda water with 2 teaspoons of syrup before serving. Add ice and a dash of basil on the top
   Nutritional Information: Calories 324; Carbs 23g; Fat 17g; Protein 0.2g

Raspberry Mocktail

Prep time: 10 minutes
Cooking time: 0 minutes
Servings: 1
Ingredients:

- 4 raspberries
- 5 mint leaves
- 2 tbsp maple syrup
- Ice, as needed
- ¼ cup raspberry juice
- 2 tbsp lime juice
- ½ cup soda water

Instructions:

1. In a large glass or jam jar, combine the raspberries, mint, and 2 tablespoons of the simple syrup.

2.Crush the components with the back of a wooden spoon. The mint leaves should not be totally broken up.

3.The glass should be filled with soda water after adding ice and lime juice. Serve.

Nutritional Information: Calories 135; Carbs 36.6g; Fat 0.3g; Protein 0.2g

Electrolyte Refresher

Prep time: 10 minutes
Cooking time: 0 minutes
Servings: 2
Ingredients:

- 1 ½ cups water
- ½ lemon, juice
- Pinch of salt
- 2 tbsp raw honey

Instructions:

1. In a big jar, combine all the ingredients. If not consumed right away, keep chilled.

Nutritional Information: Calories 67; Carbs 18.5g; Fat 0g; Protein 0g

Strawberry Lemonade

Prep time: 10 minutes
Cooking time: 0 minutes
Servings: 2
Ingredients:

- 1 ½ cups lemon-flavored tea
- ¾ cup frozen strawberries
- 1 tbsp lemon juice, fresh
- 1 tbsp maple syrup
- ½ cup ice cubes, optional

Instructions:

1. Brew the tea the previous evening and let it cool.
2. In a blender, combine the tea, strawberries, sugar, and lemon juice. When you reach the required consistency, keep adding ice cubes.
3. Add extra strawberries, lemon juice, or sugar until the ideal flavor. Pour into glasses, then add ice and strawberry slices as garnish.
   Nutritional Information: Calories 49; Carbs 12.5g; Fat 0g; Protein 0.5g

Cranberry Lemonade

Prep time: 10 minutes
Cooking time: 0 minutes
Servings: 4

Ingredients:

- 4 cups cranberries
- 2 lemons, juiced
- 1 cup basil, chopped
- 4 cups soda water for serving (optional)
- Ice for serving

Instructions:

1. Blend the cranberries, lemon juice, and basil until well combined.
2. If preferred, top with soda water and serve over ice.
   Nutritional Information: Calories 74; Carbs 18g; Fat 0.5g; Protein 2g

Mock Piña Colada

Prep time: 10 minutes + chilling time
Cooking time: 10 minutes
Servings: 4

Ingredients:

- 1 ½ cups water
- 1/3 cup sugar
- ½ cup coconut milk, canned
- 1 cup banana, frozen
- 1 tsp vanilla extract
- 1 cup fresh pineapple, cubed
- 3 cups ice
- Mint leaves for serving

Instructions:

1. Combine the sugar and water in a saucepan and heat until boiling. Once it has boiled, take it off the heat and put it in a jar in the refrigerator.
2. In a blender, combine the coconut milk, sugar water, frozen banana, vanilla bean paste, and pineapple. Blend the colada mixture until it has a smooth texture.
3. Fill a large glass with crushed ice and add the colada

   mix. Garnish with a mint leaf.
   Nutritional Information: Calories 207; Carbs 37.6g; Fat 6.9g; Protein 1.5g

Spiced Hot Chocolate

Prep time: 10 minutes

Cooking time: 5 minutes

Servings: 2

Ingredients:

- 2 cups lactose-free milk or other approved milk
- ¼ cup dark chocolate
- ½ tbsp cocoa powder
- 4 tsp brown sugar
- ½ tsp vanilla extract
- 1 tsp cinnamon, ground
- 2 tsp cornstarch
- 2 tbsp water
- Pinch dried chili flakes, optional

Instructions:

1. Warm the milk, cocoa powder, sugar, cinnamon, vanilla, and optional sprinkle of red pepper flakes in a saucepan over medium heat.
2. If the mixture is too thin, stir in the corn flour after dissolving it in cold water. Reheat and thicken the mixture by placing it back over the heat. Serve.
   Nutritional Information: Calories 349; Carbs 49g; Fat 15.5g; Protein 3.7g

Cinnamon and Cranberry Fizz

Prep time: 10 minutes

Cooking time: 0 minutes

Servings: 1

Ingredients:

- 1 tbsp cranberry juice
- Pinch of cinnamon
- ½ cup sugar-free ginger ale, ginger beer, or ginger soda water
- maple syrup, to taste

Instructions:

1. Pour the cranberry juice, cinnamon, and mix in a large glass.
2. Pour your ginger beverage into the glass and add maple syrup for desired sweetness. Serve.
   Nutritional Information: Calories 48; Carbs 12g; Fat 1g; Protein 1g

Golden Coffee

Prep time: 10 minutes

Cooking time: 5 minutes

Servings: 1

Ingredients:

- ½ tsp turmeric, ground
- ¼ tsp ginger, ground
- ¼ tsp cinnamon, ground
- ½ tsp black pepper, ground
- ¾ cup brewed coffee, decaffeinated
- ¼ cup coconut milk
- ½ tbsp honey

Instructions:

1. Add the items to a blender and blend well.
2. In a stovetop saucepan, heat thoroughly. Serve.

   Nutritional Information: Calories 189; Carbs 17g; Fat 8g; Protein 5g

White Matcha Latte

Prep time: 10 minutes
Cooking time: 5 minutes
Servings: 1
Ingredients:
- 1 ½ cups almond milk
- 1 tbsp coconut oil
- 1 bag matcha powder of choice
- ½ tsp vanilla extract

Instructions:
1. The milk and coconut oil should be combined in a pot set over medium heat. Make sure all the oil has melted.
2. Combine all the ingredients in a blender and blend until the mixture is smooth and just beginning to bubble.
   Nutritional Information: Calories 178; Carbs 1g; Fat 17g; Protein 2g

Hot Oat Milk

Prep time: 10 minutes

Cooking time: 10 minutes

Servings: 4

Ingredients:

- 1 cup rolled oats, uncooked
- 4 cups cold water
- 1 tbsp maple syrup
- 1 tsp vanilla extract

Instructions:

1. Mix the oats, water, maple syrup, and vanilla in a blender for 25 seconds. Do not over-blend.
2. Strain the mixture through cheesecloth into a sealed jar. Do not squeeze the cloth. Serve.

   Nutritional Information: Calories 226; Carbs 33.6g; Fat 5.2g; Protein 5.4g

Fruity Mimosa

Prep time: 10 minutes
Cooking time: 2 minutes
Servings: 8
Ingredients:
- ¼ cup brown sugar
- ¼ cup white sugar
- ¾ cup water
- 1 cup strawberries, fresh, chopped
- 1 bottle of sparkling wine

Instructions:
1. For 1-2 minutes on medium heat, dissolve sugar in water; let cool in the refrigerator.
2. Smoothly blend the strawberries with the sugar syrup. Add sparkling wine on top of 2 teaspoons of the mixture in a champagne glass.
   Calories 133; Carbs 18.1; Fat 0.1g; Protein 0.2g

Nutty Banana Smoothie

Prep time: 5 minutes
Cooking time: 0 minutes
Servings: 2

Ingredients:

- 2 tbsp almond butter
- 1 tsp maple syrup
- ½ cup coconut milk
- 1 frozen, unripe banana
- 1 cup lactose-free milk
- 1/3 tsp pure vanilla extract

Instructions:

1. Use a blender to thoroughly combine all the ingredients. Dispense and savor!

Nutritional Information: Calories: 194; Carbs: 14g; Fat: 12g; Protein: 11g

Cranberry Orange Smoothie

Prep time: 10 minutes
Cooking time: 5 minutes
Servings: 2

Ingredients:
- 1 1/8 cups orange juice, freshly squeezed
- 1 cup cranberries, raw
- ¼ cup almond milk, unsweetened
- 1 medium banana
- 1 tbsp lemon juice
- 1 tsp pure maple syrup
- 1 cup of ice cubes

Instructions:
1. Use a blender to thoroughly combine all the ingredients. Dispense and savor!
   Nutritional Information: Calories: 164; Carbs: 38g; Fat: 1g; Protein: 3g

Raspberry Smoothie

Prep time: 5 minutes
Cooking time: 0 minutes
Servings: 2
Ingredients:
- 1 cup raspberries
- 1 1/2 cup lactose-free milk
- 1 tsp honey
- 1/3 cup ice cubes

Instructions:

1. Use a blender to thoroughly combine all the ingredients. Dispense and savor!

Nutritional Information: Calories: 114; Carbs: 17g; Fat: 10g; Protein: 3g

Blueberry Lime Coconut Smoothie

Prep time: 5 minutes

Cooking time: 0 minutes

Servings: 1

Ingredients:

- ½ cup fresh or frozen blueberries
- 2 tbsp flaked coconut
- 2 tbsp fresh lime juice
- 4 oz lactose-free yogurt
- 1 tsp chia seeds
- 1 cup ice

Instructions:

1.Use a blender to thoroughly combine all the ingredients. Dispense and savor!

Nutritional Information: Calories 120; Carbs 17g; Fat 1g; Protein 12.2g

Strawberry Smoothie

Prep time: 5 minutes
Cooking time: 0 minutes
Servings: 1
Ingredients:

- ½ cup coconut milk
- 1 can of fresh strawberries
- ¼ cup vanilla soy ice cream
- 1 ½ tsp rice protein powder
- 1 tsp chia seeds
- ½ tbsp maple syrup
- 1 tsp lemon juice
- 6 ice cubes

Instructions:

1.Use a blender to thoroughly combine all the ingredients. Dispense and savor!

Nutritional Information: Calories 168; Carbs 21.4g; Fat 4.1g; Protein 13.9g

Pineapple Turmeric Smoothie

Prep time: 5 minutes
Cooking time: 0 minutes
Servings: 1
Ingredients:
- 1 cup of coconut water
- 1 cup chopped pineapple
- 1/2 tsp ground turmeric
- 1/2 tsp ground cinnamon
- 1/4 tsp freshly ground black pepper
- 1 tbsp chia seeds
- 1 tbsp shredded unsweetened coconut
- 1/4 tsp freshly grated ginger root
- 1/2 medium lime, peeled, seeds removed

Instructions:
1.Use a blender to thoroughly combine all the ingredients. Dispense and savor!
Nutritional Information: Calories: 225; Carbs: 53g; Fat: 6g; Protein: 3g

Berry Banana Spinach Smoothie

Prep time: 5 minutes
Cooking time: 0 minutes
Servings: 2

Ingredients:

- 1 cup rice milk
- 1 cup packed baby spinach leaves
- 1 medium firm banana
- 1/3 cup frozen strawberries
- 1/3 cup frozen blueberries
- 1/3 cup frozen raspberries

Instructions:

1.Use a blender to thoroughly combine all the ingredients. Dispense and savor!

Nutritional Information: Calories: 194; Carbs: 40g; Fat: 3g, Protein: 6g

Peanut Butter Green Smoothie

Prep time: 5 minutes
Cooking time: 0 minutes
Servings: 2
Ingredients:
- 2 cups kale (2 leaves)
- 1 cup rice milk
- 1 tbsp raw cacao powder
- 1 tbsp natural peanut butter
- 1 firm medium banana

Instructions:
1.Use a blender to thoroughly combine all the ingredients. Dispense and savor!

Nutritional Information: Calories: 205; Carbs: 31g; Fat: 7g; Protein: 9g

Strawberry Banana Smoothie

Prep time: 5 minutes
Cooking time: 0 minutes
Servings: 1

Ingredients:

- 4 strawberries
- 2/3 unripe Banana
- 6 oz pineapple juice
- 1 tsp collagen
- 1 tbsp coconut oil

Instructions:

1. Use a blender to thoroughly combine all the ingredients. Dispense and savor!

Nutritional Information: Calories: 319; Carbs: 43.6g; Fat: 14.2g; Protein: 7.8g

Banana Chia Blueberry Smoothie

Prep time: 5 minutes
Cooking time: 0 minutes
Servings: 1
Ingredients:

- 1/3 banana, peeled
- 10 blueberries
- ½ cup spinach
- ¼ cup ice cubes
- 2 tbsp chia seeds
- ½ cup unsweetened almond milk

Instructions:

1. Use a blender to thoroughly combine all the ingredients. Dispense and savor!

Nutritional Information: Calories: 517; Carbs: 22g; Fat: 8.9g; Protein: 9.6g

Cinnamon Carrot Milkshake

Prep time: 5 minutes
Cooking time: 0 minutes
Servings: 1
Ingredients:

- ¼ cup collagen
- ¼ tsp turmeric
- ½ cup coconut cream
- ½ tsp cinnamon
- 1 tbsp maple syrup
- ¼ tsp ginger powder
- ½ cup unsweetened coconut milk
- 2 cups carrots, peeled, chopped, & cooked

Instructions:

1. Use a blender to thoroughly combine all the ingredients. Dispense and savor!

Nutritional Information: Calories: 249; Carbs: 23.2g; Fat: 17.4g; Protein: 3.1g

Berries and Sea Moss Smoothie

Prep time: 5 minutes
Cooking time: 0 minutes
Servings: 2
Ingredients:
- 1 cup coconut water
- 2 cups lettuce leaves
- 1 banana, peeled
- 1 cup berries, mixed
- 1 tbsp sea moss
- 2 key limes, juiced

Instructions:

1. Use a blender to thoroughly combine all the ingredients. Dispense and savor!

Nutritional Information: Calories: 163; Carbs: 35g; Fat: 0.9g; Protein: 3.7g

Raspberry and Chard Smoothie

Prep time: 5 minutes

Cooking time: 0 minutes

Servings: 2

Ingredients:

- 2 cups coconut water
- 2 cups Swiss chards
- 2 key limes, juiced
- 2 cups fresh whole raspberries

Instructions:

1. Use a blender to thoroughly combine all the ingredients. Dispense and savor!

Nutritional Information: Calories: 137; Carbs: 27g; Fat: 1.4g; Protein: 3.4g

Berries and Kale Smoothie

Prep time: 5 minutes
Cooking time: 0 minutes
Servings: 2
Ingredients:
- 1 cup of spring water
- 1 cup berries, mixed
- 2 cups kale leaves, fresh

Instructions:
1. Use a blender to thoroughly combine all the ingredients. Dispense and savor!
Nutritional Information: Calories: 112; Carbs :24.4g; Fat: 0.7g; Protein: 2g

Blueberry Lime Smoothie

Prep time: 5 minutes
Cooking time: 0 minutes
Servings: 1
Ingredients:

- ½ cup blueberries, fresh or frozen
- 2 tbsp coconut flakes
- 2 tbsp lime juice, fresh
- ½ cup Greek or lactose-free yogurt
- 1 tsp chia seeds
- 2 tbsp water
- Ice, as needed

Instructions:

1. Use a blender to thoroughly combine all the ingredients. Dispense and savor!

Nutritional Information: Calories: 319; Carbs :26g; Fat: 23g; Protein: 7g

Blueberry, Kiwi, and Mint Smoothie

Prep time: 5 minutes
Cooking time: 0 minutes
Servings: 1
Ingredients:

- ½ cup blueberries, frozen
- 1 kiwi, small, peeled
- 1/3 cup Greek yogurt
- 1/3 cup water
- 6 mint leaves, fresh

Instructions:

1.Use a blender to thoroughly combine all the ingredients. Dispense and savor!

Nutritional Information: Calories: 226; Carbs :27g; Fat: 12g; Protein: 6g

Fruit Salad Smoothie

Prep time: 5 minutes

Cooking time: 0 minutes

Servings: 2

Ingredients:

- 1 cup canned fruit salad, frozen
- 2 tbsp lactose-free yogurt
- 2 tbsp coconut milk
- 2 tsp coconut, shredded
- 2 tsp walnuts, chopped finely
- 1 tsp lemon zest, optional
- ½ cup water to thin out the mixture

Instructions:

1. In a blender, puree everything except the walnuts and coconut shreds until smooth.
2. Before serving, sprinkle walnuts and coconut flakes on top.
   Nutritional Information: Calories: 129; Carbs :15g; Fat: 8g; Protein: 2g

Orange Banana Alkaline Smoothie

Prep time: 5 minutes
Cooking time: 0 minutes
Servings: 2
Ingredients:

- ½ cup coconut water
- 1 cup water
- 2 medium bananas
- 4 oranges, peeled
- ¼ tsp bromide plus powder
- 2 tsp light-colored agave syrup

Instructions:

1. Use a blender to thoroughly combine all the ingredients. Dispense and savor!

Nutritional Information: Calories: 126; Carbs: 31g; Fat: 1g; Protein: 2g

Melon Cucumber Smoothie

Prep time: 5 minutes

Cooking time: 0 minutes

Servings: 2

Ingredients:

- 1 cup melon, peeled & chopped into bits
- 1 medium-sized cucumber, chopped into bits
- 2 tbsp lime juice
- 2 cups water

Instructions:

1. Use a blender to thoroughly combine all the ingredients. Dispense and savor!

Nutritional Information: Calories: 82; Carbs: 20g; Fat: 1g; Protein: 2g

Oatmeal Cookie Breakfast Smoothie

Prep time: 5 minutes
Cooking time: 0 minutes
Servings: 1
Ingredients:

- 1 banana, peeled & sliced
- ¾ cup almond milk
- ¼ cup ice
- 1/8 tbsp vanilla
- ½ tsp cinnamon powder
- 2 tbsp rolled oats
- A dash of ground nutmeg

Instructions:

1. Use a blender to thoroughly combine all the ingredients. Dispense and savor!

Nutritional Information: Calories 303; Carbs 52.1g; Fat 7.8g; Protein 5.5g

Almond Butter Smoothie

Prep time: 5 minutes

Cooking time: 0 minutes

Servings: 2

Ingredients:

- 3 cups almond milk, unsweetened
- 12 ice cubes
- ¼ tsp pure almond extract, sugar-free
- 1 tbsp. ground cinnamon
- ¼ cup flax meal
- 30 drops Stevia sweetener, liquid
- ¼ cup almond butter, unsalted and softened

Instructions:

1. Use a blender to thoroughly combine all the ingredients. Dispense .

Nutritional Information: Calories: 344; Carbs: 24g; Fat: 24g; Protein: 14g

Green Kiwi Smoothie

Prep time: 5 minutes
Cooking time: 0 minutes
Servings: 2

Ingredients:

- 1 cup seedless green grapes
- 1 kiwi, peeled & chopped
- 2 tbsp water
- 8 inches cucumber, cut into chunks
- 2 cups baby spinach
- 1 ½ cups ice cubes

Instructions:

1. Use a blender to thoroughly combine all the ingredients. Dispense and savor!

Nutritional Information: Calories 132; Carbs 33g; Fat 1g; Protein 3g

Pumpkin Smoothie

Prep time: 5 minutes
Cooking time: 0 minutes
Servings: 1
Ingredients:
- ½ frozen medium ripe bananas, peeled and sliced
- ¼ cup pumpkin puree
- ½ cup coconut milk
- ¼ tsp pumpkin pie spice
- 1 tbsp maple syrup
- ½ cup crushed ice
- A pinch of cinnamon

Instructions:
1. Use a blender to thoroughly combine all the ingredients. Dispense and savor!
Nutritional Information: Calories 695; Carbs 52.3g; Fat 37.7g; Protein 14.3g

Chocolate Sesame Smoothie

Prep time: 5 minutes
Cooking time: 0 minutes
Servings: 1

Ingredients:

- 1 tbsp sesame seeds
- 2 tsp unsweetened raw cocoa powder
- 1/2 medium banana, peeled and sliced
- Flesh from 1/8 slice of avocado
- 1 tbsp maple syrup
- 1 cup coconut milk
- ½ cup ice

Instructions:

1. Use a blender to thoroughly combine all the ingredients. Dispense and savor!

Nutritional Information: Calories 406; Carbs 57.3g; Fat 17.5g; Protein 11.8g

Basic Recipes

Balsamic Vinaigrette

Prep time: 5 min
Serves: 10
Difficulty: Moderate
Ingredients

- ¼ cup garlic-infused extra-virgin olive oil
- ¼ cup balsamic vinegar
- 1 teaspoon sugar
- ½ teaspoon salt
- ¼ teaspoon freshly ground black pepper

Instructions:

1. In a small mixing bowl, whisk the oil, vinegar, sugar, salt, and pepper until the sugar and salt are dissolved. Serve immediately or cover and refrigerate for up to four days.
   Nutritional Information: Calories: 82kcal |Fat: 0.1 g| Protein: 0.2g |Carbohydrates: 3.8 g.

Blue Cheese Dressing

Prep time: 5 min
Serves: 12
Difficulty: Moderate

Ingredients

- ⅓ cup crumbled Gorgonzola cheese
- ⅓ cup mayonnaise
- ⅓ cup lactose-free sour cream
- 1 tablespoon fresh lemon juice

Instructions:

1. In a small dish, stir together the cheese, mayonnaise, sour cream, and lemon juice. Cover tightly with plastic wrap and chill until ready to serve.

   Nutritional Information: Calories: 64kcal| Fat 1.8g|Protein 0.4g| Carbohydrate 1g

Smoky Ranch Dressing

Prep time: 5 min
Serves: 10-18
Difficulty: Moderate
Ingredients

- ¼ cup mayonnaise
- ¼ cup lactose-free sour cream
- 1 tablespoon garlic-infused olive oil
- 2 tablespoons fresh lime juice
- 1 teaspoon sugar
- ½ teaspoon salt
- ¼ teaspoon sweet smoked paprika
- 1 teaspoon chia seeds (optional)

Instructions:

1. In a small mixing bowl, combine the mayonnaise, sour cream, oil, lime juice, sugar, salt, paprika, and seeds, if using. Stir until thoroughly combined. Carefully cover and chill for 30 minutes before serving.
Nutritional Information: Calories: 71kcal| Fat 2g|Protein 0.5g| Carbohydrate 2g

Lemon French Dressing

Prep time: 5 min

Serves: 12

Difficulty: Moderate

Ingredients

- ¼ cup fresh lemon juice
- 3 tablespoons olive oil
- 1 tablespoon garlic-infused olive oil
- ½ teaspoon salt
- ½ teaspoon dry mustard
- ½ teaspoon sweet paprika
- 1 ½ teaspoons sugar

Instructions:

1. In a blender or small bowl, combine the lemon juice, oils, salt, mustard, paprika, and sugar and blend until smooth. Serve immediately.

   Nutritional Information: Calories: 82kcal|Fat 1g| Protein 0g|Carbohydrates 7.2g

Basil Pesto

Prep time: 5 min
Serves: 12
Difficulty: Moderate

Ingredients

- ¼ cup water
- ½ cup pine nuts
- 1 garlic-infused olive oil
- 4 cups tightly packed fresh basil
- 1 cup grated Parmesan cheese
- 1 ½ teaspoons salt

Instructions:

1. In a food processor or blender, pulse the water and pine nuts until the nuts are broken down into tiny pieces. While the blades are moving on medium-high, add the oil and basil alternately, in thirds, and process until the mixture is uniform and has the consistency of sand. Use the tamper that is included with your blender to push the basil leaves as necessary closer to the blades. Salt and Parmesan cheese are added while mixing at a low speed.

2. Store the pesto in the refrigerator tightly wrapped or freeze individual servings for later use; ice cube trays or 12-pint canning jars are great for this.
   Nutritional Information: Calories: 78kcal| Fat 1.5g|Protein 0.3g| Carbohydrate 1.2g

Cilantro-Chile-Mint Pesto

Prep time: 5 min

Serves: 5

Difficulty: Moderate

Ingredients

- 1 small fresh green or red chili, chopped
- 1 tablespoon minced fresh ginger
- 2 tablespoons water
- 3 tablespoons fresh lime juice (from I large lime)
- 2 tablespoons walnut pieces
- ¼ cup olive oil
- 1 teaspoon sugar
- 1 teaspoon salt
- 2 cups tightly packed fresh cilantro leaves
- 1 cup tightly packed fresh mint leaves

Instructions:

1. In a food processor or blender, combine the chili, ginger, water, lime juice, walnuts, oil, sugar, and salt. Purée until smooth. While the blender is running, open the lid's hole and cram handfuls of cilantro and mint leaves inside; you may need to cover the lid's hole with your hand between additions of leaves to avoid spilling. Process until you have a coarse paste. If desired, freeze in little pieces or chill until ready to serve.

Nutritional Information: Calories: 86kcal|Fat:5g|Carbohydrate:2g|Protein: 1.2g

Beef Stock

Prep time: 50 min
Serves: 12
Difficulty: Moderate

Ingredients

- 1 small onion, quartered
- 1 garlic clove
- 2 tablespoons olive oil
- 10 cups water and/or pan drippings
- 2 carrots, coarsely chopped
- 1 bay leaf
- 10 whole peppercorns
- 1 teaspoon salt
- 1 tablespoon reduced-sodium soy sauce

Instructions:

1. . Set the oven's temperature to 400 degrees Fahrenheit. Roast the beef bones in a roasting pan for an hour.
2. Over medium heat, sauté the onion and garlic in the olive oil in a big stockpot. When the onion and garlic are translucent, remove them from the saucepan and put them away for later use. Keep the flavored oil in the pot.
3. Add the carrots, water, bay leaf, peppercorns, salt, and soy sauce along with the beef bones, drippings, or water, and all of the other ingredients. Over high heat, bring to a boil; then, decrease heat to a low setting, cover, and simmer for 112 to 2 hours, or until the stock has reduced by about 20%. Skim any foam from the surface as necessary.
4. After the stock has cooled to a safe temperature to handle, use a slotted spoon or a sieve to sift out the bones and other solids. Take out the solids, then discard them. Use

immediately, cover and refrigerate for up to three days, or freeze for up to three months. Once the stock has cooled, the hard fat on top may be easily removed, if desired.

Nutritional Information: Calories: 152kcal| Fat 7g|Protein 12g| Carbohydrates 2.9g

Chicken Stock

Prep time: 5 min
Serves: 12
Difficulty: Moderate

Ingredients

- 1 small onion, quartered
- 1 garlic clove
- 2 tablespoons olive oil
- 1 carcass from a roasted chicken, including bones and skin
- 2 large carrots, coarsely chopped
- 10 cups water and/or pan drippings
- 1 bay leaf
- 10 whole peppercorns
- 1 teaspoon salt
- 1 tablespoon reduced-sodium soy sauce

Instructions:

1. Over medium heat, sauté the onion and garlic in the olive oil in a big stockpot. When the onion and garlic are translucent, remove them from the saucepan and put them aside, keeping the flavored oil in the pot.
2. Fill the saucepan with water, drippings, carrots, a bay leaf, peppercorns, salt, and soy sauce. Over high heat, bring to a boil; then, decrease heat to a low setting, cover, and simmer for 112 to 2 hours, or until the stock has reduced by about 20%.
3. Let the stock cool fully before filtering or using a slotted spoon to remove the solids. Take out the solids, then discard them. Use immediately, cover and refrigerate for up to three days, or freeze for up to three months. If desired, the

hardened fat may be easily removed once the stock has cooled.

Nutritional Information: Calories: 123kcal| Fat 2g| Protein 8g| Carbohydrate 6g

Seasoned Salt

Prep time: 5 min
Serves: 30
Difficulty: Moderate
Ingredients

- 1 tablespoon medium salt crystals
- 1 tablespoon black peppercorns
- 1 tablespoon coriander seeds
- 1 tablespoon mustard seeds
- 1 teaspoon red pepper flakes

Instructions:

1. In a small bowl, mix the salt, peppercorns, seeds, and red pepper flakes. The combination should fill a pepper mill or grinder halfway. Serve at the table with your favorite meals topped with fresh, seasoned salt, if you'd like.

   Nutritional Information: Calories: 12kcal| Fat 0g|Proteins 0g |Carbohydrates 0.5g

Taco Seasoning Mix

Prep time: 5 min
Serves: 32
Difficulty: Moderate
Ingredients

- ¼ cup cornstarch
- ¼ cup ground ancho chili
- ¼ cup ground ancho chili
- 2 tablespoons ground cumin
- 1 teaspoon sweet smoked paprika
- 2 teaspoons salt

Instructions:

1. Combine the cornstarch, salt, cumin, paprika, and ground chili in an airtight container. Although taco seasoning mix may be kept indefinitely, it tastes best when used within six months.
   Nutritional Information: Calories: 16kcal| Fat 0.2g|Protein 0g| Carbohydrate 3g

Garlic -Infused Olive Oil

Prep time: 20 min
Serves: 12
Difficulty: Moderate
 Ingredients

- 1 cup plus 1 teaspoon extra-virgin olive oil
- 8 garlic cloves

Instructions:

1. In a small, heavy saucepan, boil the oil and garlic over medium heat until the garlic begins to crackle and little bubbles rise steadily to the top. Cook for 10 minutes, or until the garlic is tender, over low heat.
2. After letting it cool for a few minutes, remove the garlic and carefully bottle the oil before keeping it in the fridge for up to 4 days.
   Nutritional Information: Calories: 98kcal|Fat 2g|Protein 0g| Carbohydrate 2g

Zippy Ketchup

Prep time: 5 min
Serves: 12
Difficulty: Moderate
Ingredients

- 1 14.5-ounce can diced tomatoes
- 1 tablespoon garlic-infused olive oil
- 1 small red chili, fresh or dried, minced
- ⅓ cup sugar
- ⅓ cup apple cider vinegar
- ¼ teaspoon sweet smoked paprika
- ¼ teaspoon ground allspice
- ⅛ teaspoon ground cloves
- ½ teaspoon salt, or more as needed

Instructions:

1. In a 3-quart saucepan, combine the tomatoes, juices, oil, chili, sugar, vinegar, spices, and salt. Over medium-high heat, bring the mixture to a boil. Then, reduce the heat to low and simmer the mixture, uncovered, for one hour.
2. Turn off the heat and let the pot cool for 30 minutes, or until the ketchup is secure enough to handle. In a blender, puree the ketchup until it is absolutely smooth.
3. Store the ketchup in the refrigerator for up to 4 days or in the freezer for 2 to 3 months.
   Nutritional Information: Calories: 97kcal| Fat 2g |Protein 1.2g| Carbohydrate 8g

Marinara Sauce

Prep time: 35 min
Serves: 10
Difficulty: Moderate

Ingredients

- 4 tablespoons olive oil or garlic-infused olive oil
- 4 tablespoons olive oil or garlic-infused olive oil
- 1 bunch scallions (green parts only), thinly sliced
- 1 28-ounce can be crushed or finely chopped tomatoes
- 1 14.5-ounce can crush or finely chopped tomatoes
- ½ teaspoon salt, or more as needed
- 1 tablespoon dried basil
- 1 tablespoon dried oregano
- 1 tablespoon sugar

Instructions:

1. In a 4-quart saucepan with the oil on medium heat, sauté the scallion greens for three minutes. Add the tomatoes and their juices, as well as the salt, sugar, basil, and oregano. Serve right away, or closely cover and store in the refrigerator for up to 4 days. Bring the sauce to a boil, covered, over medium-high heat; then, reduce the heat to low and simmer for approximately 30 minutes.
Nutritional Information: Calories: 79kcal| Fat 0g|Protein 1.8g| Carbohydrate 10.9g

Spicy Peanut Sauce

Prep time: 5 min

Serves: 7

Difficulty: Moderate

Ingredients

- 6 tablespoons natural peanut butter
- 2 tablespoons reduced-sodium soy sauce
- ½ cup canned coconut milk
- 1 tablespoon minced fresh ginger
- 2 teaspoons sugar
- 1 teaspoon toasted or spicy sesame oil

Instructions:

1. In a medium bowl, combine the peanut butter, soy sauce, coconut milk, ginger, sugar, and sesame oil. Whisk until well combined the peanut butter, soy sauce, coconut milk, ginger, sugar, and sesame oil. Whisk until well combined. As soon as you can, serve.
2. Store any leftovers in the refrigerator for up to 4 days in an airtight container; thaw before serving.
   Nutritional Information: Calories: 85 kcal| Carbohydrate 6g | Fat 2.5g | Protein 1g

Pineapple -Teriyaki Sauce

Prep time: 5 min

Serves: 7

Difficulty: Moderate

Ingredients

- ¼ cup reduced-sodium soy sauce
- ½ cup crushed pineapple, with juice
- 1 tablespoon toasted or spicy sesame oil
- 1 tablespoon garlic-infused olive oil
- 1 tablespoon rice vinegar
- 1 tablespoon minced fresh ginger
- 2 tablespoons light brown sugar
- ¼ teaspoon red pepper flakes (optional)

Instructions:

1. In a large glass or ceramic dish, combine the soy sauce, pineapple, pineapple juice, oils, vinegar, ginger, brown sugar, and red pepper flakes. Put the steak, fish, or chicken in the marinade and let it sit in the fridge for up to 10 hours. Alternatively, you may pour the marinade into a zip-top bag and let it sit there.

2. Drain the marinade from the meat, fish, or poultry and heat the grill. When the marinade has decreased and thickened somewhat, transfer it to a small saucepan, bring to a boil, and simmer for 2 to 3 minutes. Brush the marinade over the meat, fish, or poultry numerous times while grilling. Any leftover marinade must be thrown away.
Nutritional Information: Calories: 55kcal| Fat 1.8g|Protein 1g| Carbohydrate 6g

Sourdough Bread Croutons

Prep time: 45 min
Serves: 12
Difficulty: Moderate

Ingredients

- 2 tablespoons melted butter
- 2 tablespoons extra-virgin olive oil
- 5 cups stale sourdough bread, cut into ½-inch cubes
- ¼ teaspoon salt
- ¼ teaspoon freshly ground black pepper
- ¼ teaspoon poultry seasoning

Instructions:

1. In a large mixing bowl, toss the bread cubes with the melted butter and oil and preheat the oven to 250 degrees Fahrenheit. Mix thoroughly after uniformly seasoning the bread pieces with salt, pepper, and chicken spice.

2. Spread the bread cubes evenly over two greased baking sheets and bake for 20 minutes. After stirring, put the pans back in the oven for an additional 20 minutes. After turning off the oven and opening the door a little, let the bread cubes cool to room temperature.

3. After the cubes have cooled, place them in a tightly covered container. Make sure the cooled croutons are completely dry before storing them to prevent mold.
   Nutritional Information: Calories: 164kcal| Fat 1.8g|Protein 2g| Carbohydrate 17g

Toasted Bread Crumbs

Prep time: 25min
Serves: 22
Difficulty: Moderate

Ingredients

- 1 Bread loaf

Instructions:

1. Set the oven's temperature to 250 degrees Fahrenheit. On top of an ungreased cookie sheet, arrange the bread slices in a single layer on a wire rack. The bread does not need to brown; it just needs to be cooked for approximately 20 minutes or until it is dry. Once the oven is off and the door is propped open, let the bread cool to room temperature. With your hands, tear the bread slices into 2-inch pieces. Grind the bread in small batches in a blender or food processor until it resembles coarse sand.
2. Before keeping the breadcrumbs in an airtight container for up to a month, thoroughly chill them to prevent mold growth. **Nutritional Information:** Calories: 78kcal| Fat 0.8g|Protein 0.2g| Carbohydrate 18g

Salsa Verde

Prep time: 15 min
Serves: 1
Difficulty: Moderate
Ingredients

- 2 handfuls of flat-leaf parsley, rinsed and dried
- 3 anchovy fillets in oil, drained (optional)
- 2 teaspoons capers, rinsed and drained
- 1 tablespoon garlic-infused olive oil
- 2 tablespoons olive oil
- 2 tablespoons fresh lemon juice, or to taste
- Salt and freshly ground black pepper

Instructions:

1. Pulse the parsley, capers, and anchovy fillets (if using) in a food processor or blender until smooth.
2. Drizzle the olive oil and garlic-infused oil in small amounts, carefully combining after each addition.
3. Add the lemon juice and season with salt and pepper to taste. For up to 5 days, put in a dish or jar, cover, and store in the fridge.
   Nutritional Information: Calories: 53kcal| Fat 1g|Protein 0.2g| Carbohydrates 1.9g

Basil Pesto

Prep time: 45 min
Serves: 1
Difficulty: Moderate
Ingredients

- 2 handfuls of basil leaves, rinsed and dried
- 2 tablespoons garlic-infused olive oil
- 2 tablespoons olive oil, plus more as needed
- 1/3 cup pine nuts
- 1/3 cup grated Parmesan
- Salt and freshly ground black pepper

Instructions:

1. Combine the basil, garlic-infused oil, olive oil, pine nuts, and Parmesan until thoroughly combined in a food processor or blender.
2. To taste, add salt and pepper to the food.
3. Add additional oil if you want a more liquid pesto for drizzling. spoon into a dish or jar and cover with a thin layer of olive oil.
4. After covering, store in the fridge for up to 5 days or in the freezer for up to 2 months.
Nutritional Information: Calories: 102 kcal|Fat 2.6g|Protein 1.3g| Carbohydrate 7g

Sun-Dried Tomato Spread

Prep time: 20 min
Serves: 1
Difficulty: Moderate
Ingredients

- 1 cup sun-dried tomatoes in oil, drained, and roughly chopped (oil reserved)
- 1⁄4 cup roughly chopped flat-leaf parsley
- 2 heaping tablespoons reduced-fat cream cheese, at room temperature
- 1 tablespoon garlic-infused olive oil
- 3 tablespoons olive oil
- Salt and freshly ground black pepper

Instructions:

1. Sun-dried tomatoes, preserved oil, parsley, and cream cheese should all be well combined in a food processor or blender.
2. Once the mixture is almost smooth, gradually add the garlic-infused oil and olive oil.
3. Add salt and pepper to taste when seasoning.
4. Put in a container or jar, cover, and store chilled for up to three days.
Nutritional Information: Calories: 134kcal|Carbohydrate 3g| Fat 5.5g|Protein 2g

Olive Tapenade

Prep time: 20 min
Serves: 1
Difficulty: Moderate

Ingredients

- 1 cup pitted black olives
- 1 1/2 ounces anchovy fillets in oil, drained
- 2 heaping tablespoons gluten-free mayonnaise
- 2 teaspoons garlic-infused olive oil
- 2 teaspoons olive oil
- 2 teaspoons fresh lemon juice
- Pepper to taste (optional)

Instructions:

1. Combine all of the ingredients in a food processor or blender, and process until smooth.
2. The texture of the tapenade should still be present. For up to 5 days, put in a dish or jar, cover, and store in the fridge.
   Nutritional Information: Calories: 83kcal | Fat 4.8g | Protein 0.1g | Carbohydrate 0.7g

Mango Salsa

Prep time: 10min
Serves: 6
Difficulty: Moderate
Ingredients:

- 2 ripe mangoes, peeled and diced
- 1 serrano chili, finely chopped (optional)
- 2 green onions, finely chopped
- 1/2 red pepper, finely chopped
- 1/2 yellow pepper, finely chopped
- 1cup fresh cilantro, finely chopped
- Juice of 1 lime (about 2 tablespoons), or to taste

Instructions:

1. To create a dip or guacamole accompaniment, mix the mango chunks with the chopped chilies, green onions, red and yellow bell peppers, cilantro, and lime juice in a bowl.
Nutritional Information: Calories: 64kcal |Fat 0g| Protein 0g| Carbohydrate 16g

Celery Root Tahini Dip

Prep time: 10min
Serves: 6
Difficulty: Moderate
 Ingredients:

- 1 medium celery root, skinned and chopped (about 2 cups)
- 2 tablespoons of olive oil or coconut oil
- 1/2 an onion
- 1 to 2 cloves garlic
- 1 teaspoon turmeric
- 1 /2 to 1 teaspoon sea salt
- 11 /2 teaspoons of Herbs de Provence mixture or rosemary
- 2 tablespoons tahini
- Juice of 1 /2 a lemon (about 1 /8 cup)
- 1/8 teaspoon each sea salt and pepper, or to taste

Instructions:

1. After boiling the celery root for approximately 5 minutes, or until it is tender, drain it and place it in a basin.
2. Fry the celery root, turmeric, sea salt, and herbs after frying the onions and garlic in the same oil. Cook the celery root in a gentle caramelization while stirring often.
3. In a mixing bowl, combine the tahini and lemon juice. At this point, you have the option of eating the mixture raw, mashing it with a potato masher, or blending it.
   Nutritional Information: Calories: 149kcal| Fat 2.9g|Protein 0.7g| Carbohydrate 23g

Basic Nut or Seed Pâté

Prep time: 5min
Serves: 8
Difficulty: Moderate
Ingredients:

- 2 cups of seeds or nuts (such as sunflower seeds, pumpkin seeds, almonds, macadamia nuts, or cashews)
- Juice of 3 lemons (about 3/4 cup)
- 1/4 cup of water
- 1 heaping teaspoon of sea salt
- 4 cloves garlic

Instructions:

1. Grind the nuts or seeds in a powerful blender or coffee grinder. At a time, we advise grinding a quarter cup. If you ground your coffee in a bowl, put the powdered mixture aside.
2. Blend or process the lemon juice, water, salt, and garlic in a food processor.
3. Combine the powdered mixture with the mixture of lemon juice. To get the desired consistency, you may need to add a few more tablespoons of water and lemon juice.
   Nutritional Information: Calories: 68kcal | Fat 2g|Protein 0.2g| Carbohydrate 7g

Lemon Gone Wild Dressing

Prep time: 5min

Serves: 6

Difficulty: Moderate

 Ingredients:

- 1⁄4 cup extra-virgin olive oil
- 2 tablespoons fresh lemon juice
- 3⁄4 teaspoon minced fresh garlic
- 3 ⁄4 teaspoon salt
- 1⁄8 teaspoon freshly cracked black pepper
- 3⁄4 teaspoon fresh thyme leaves

Instructions:

1. To fully blend all the ingredients and for better presentation,

    keep the vinaigrette clear (not emulsified) in a mixing bowl.
    Nutritional Information: Calories: 69kcal|Fat 1g|Protein
    0.2g| Carbohydrate 19g

Asian Dressing

Prep time: 5min
Serves: 2
Difficulty: Moderate
Ingredients:

- 1⁄4 cup sesame oil
- 4 tablespoons vegetable oil
- 1⁄4 cup soy sauce
- 1⁄4 cup rice wine vinegar
- 2 tablespoons maple syrup
- 1 tablespoon light miso paste (optional)

Instructions:

1. In a large mixing bowl, add all the ingredients and whisk well to incorporate.

Nutritional Information: Calories: 140kcal |Fat 4.2g| Protein 1g| Carbohydrate 21g

Shannon's Spicy Caesar Dressing

Prep time: 5min

Serves: 15

Difficulty: Moderate

Ingredients:

- 1 cup flaxseed, olive, or hemp oil
- Juice of 1 to 2 lemons (about 1/2 cup)
- 1/3 cup raw tahini
- 1 to 2 cloves garlic
- Nama Shoyu, or 1/2 teaspoon sea salt

Instructions:

1. Place all the ingredients in a blender and blend until completely smooth.

Nutritional Information: Calories: 165kcal |Fat 3.2g| Protein 3.4g| Carbohydrate 15g

Angela's Happy Mayo

Prep time: 10min
Serves: 2
Difficulty: Moderate

Ingredients:

- 1⁄2 cup raw tahini
- 1 to 2 tablespoons fresh lemon juice
- 2 tablespoons yacon syrup, or 6 soaked honey dates, pitted
- 1 teaspoon sea salt
- Juice of 1 orange (about 1⁄4 cup)
- 2 tablespoons fresh dill
- 1 cup water

Instructions:

1. Combine all the ingredients in a mixing dish, then either spread over a favorite sandwich or toss with your favorite salad.
   Nutritional Information: Calories: 94kcal | Fat 2.5g| Protein 0.9g| Carbohydrate 26g

Home-style Mayonnaise

Prep time: 5min
Serves: 2
Difficulty: Moderate
Ingredients:

- 1 egg
- 1 teaspoon dry mustard
- 1/2 teaspoon each white pepper and sea salt
- Pinch of cayenne pepper
- 3 tablespoons lemon juice
- 1 cup olive oil or safflower oil
- 1 tablespoon hot water

Instructions:

1. In a blender, combine the egg, mustard, white pepper, salt, cayenne pepper, and lemon juice.
   Blend until well combined.
2. Drizzle the oil in gradually while the mixer is still running.
   Nutritional Information: Calories: 182kcal | Fat 2.9g| Protein 3.4g| Carbohydrate 24g

Lightning Source UK Ltd.
Milton Keynes UK
UKHW020630300123
416164UK00012B/1857

9 781803 619637